The New Board: Changing Issues, Roles and Relationships

T0256312

The New Board: Changing Issues, Roles and Relationships has been co-published simultaneously as *Residential Treatment for Children & Youth*, Volume 16, Number 4 1999.

The *Residential Treatment for Children & Youth* Monographic "Separates"

Below is a list of "separates," which in serials librarianship means a special issue simultaneously published as a special journal issue or double-issue *and* as a "separate" hardbound monograph. (This is a format which we also call a "DocuSerial.")

"Separates" are published because specialized libraries or professionals may wish to purchase a specific thematic issue by itself in a format which can be separately cataloged and shelved, as opposed to purchasing the journal on an on-going basis. Faculty members may also more easily consider a "separate" for classroom adoption.

"Separates" are carefully classified separately with the major book jobbers so that the journal tie-in can be noted on new book order slips to avoid duplicate purchasing.

You may wish to visit Haworth's website at . . .

http://www.haworthpressinc.com

. . . to search our online catalog for complete tables of contents of these separates and related publications.

You may also call 1-800-HAWORTH (outside US/Canada: 607-722-5857), or Fax: 1-800-895-0582 (outside US/Canada: 607-771-0012), or e-mail at:

getinfo@haworthpressinc.com

The New Board: Changing Issues, Roles and Relationships, edited by Nadia Ehrlich Finkelstein, MS, ACSW, and Raymond Schimmer, MAT (Vol. 16, No. 4, 1999). *This innovative book offers very specific, real life examples and informed recommendations for board management of nonprofit residential service agencies and explains why and how to consider redesigning your board form and practice. You will explore variations of board structures, managed care pressure, increased complexity of service, reduced board member availability, and relevant theoretical discussions complete with pertinent reports on the practice of boards in the nonprofit residential service field.*

Outcome Assessment in Residential Treatment, edited by Steven I. Pfeiffer, PhD (Vol. 13, No. 4, 1996). *"Presents a logical and systematic response, based on research, to the detractors of residential treatment centers." (Canada's Children (Child Welfare League of Canada))*

Residential Education as an Option for At-Risk Youth, edited by Jerome Beker, EdD, and Douglas Magnuson, MA (Vol. 13, No. 3, 1996). *"As a remarkable leap forward, as an approach to child welfare, it is required reading for professionals–from child care workers to administrators and planners–or for anyone in search of hope for children trapped in the bitter problems of a blighted and disordered existence . . . It is instructive, practical, and humanistic." (Howard Goldstein, DSW, Professor Emeritus, Case Western Reserve University; Author, The Home on Gorham Street)*

When Love Is Not Enough: The Management of Covert Dynamics in Organizations that Treat Children and Adolescents, edited by Donna Piazza, PhD (Vol. 13, No. 1, 1996). *"Addresses the difficult question of 'unconscious dynamics' within institutions which care for children and adolescents. The subject matter makes for fascinating reading, and anyone who has had experience of residential institutions for disturbed children will find themselves nodding in agreement throughout the book." (Emotional and Behavioural Difficulties)*

Applied Research in Residential Treatment, edited by Gordon Northrup, MD (Vol. 12, No. 1, 1995). *"The authors suggest appropriate topics for research projects, give practical suggestions on design, and provide example research reports." (Reference & Research Book News)*

Managing the Residential Treatment Center in Troubled Times, edited by Gordon Northrup, MD (Vol. 11, No. 4, 1994). *"A challenging manual for a challenging decade. . . . Takes the eminently sensible position that our failures are as worthy of analysis as our successes. This approach is both sobering and instructive." (Nancy Woodruff Ment, MSW, BCD, Associate Executive Director, Julia Dyckman Andrus Memorial, Yonkers, New York)*

The Management of Sexuality in Residential Treatment, edited by Gordon Northrup, MD (Vol. 11, No. 2, 1994). *"Must reading for residential treatment center administrators and all treatment personnel." (Irving N. Berlin, MD, Emeritus Professor, School of Medicine, University of New Mexico; Clinical Director, Child & Adolescent Services, Charter Hospital of Albuquerque and Medical Director, Namaste Residential Treatment Center)*

Sexual Abuse and Residential Treatment, edited by Wander de C. Braga, MD, and Raymond Schimmer (Vol. 11, No. 1, 1994). *"Ideas are presented for assisting victims in dealing with past abuse and protecting them from future abuse in the facility." (Coalition Commentary (Illinois Coalition Against Sexual Assault))*

Milieu Therapy: Significant Issues and Innovative Applications, edited by Jerome M. Goldsmith, EdD, and Jacquelyn Sanders, PhD (Vol. 10, No. 3, 1993). *This tribute to Bruno Bettelheim illuminates continuing efforts to further understanding of the caring process and its impact upon healing and repair measures for disturbed children in residential care.*

Severely Disturbed Youngsters and the Parental Alliance, edited by Jacquelyn Sanders, PhD, and Barry L. Childress, MD (Vol. 9, No. 4, 1992). *"Establishes the importance of a therapeutic alliance with the parents of severely disturbed young people to improve the success of counseling." (Public Welfare)*

Crisis Intervention in Residential Treatment: The Clinical Innovations of Fritz Redl, edited by William C. Morse, PhD (Vol. 8, No. 4, 1991). *"Valuable in helping us set directions for continuing Redl's courageous trail-blazing work." (Reading (A Journal of Reviews and Commentary in Mental Health))*

Adolescent Suicide: Recognition, Treatment and Prevention, edited by Barry Garfinkel, MD, and Gordon Northrup, MD (Vol. 7, No. 1, 1990). *"Distills highly relevant information about the identification and treatment of suicidal adolescents into a pithy volume which will be highly accessible by all mental health professionals." (Norman E. Alessi, MD, Director, Child Diagnostic and Research Unit, The University of Michigan Medical Center)*

Psychoanalytic Approaches to the Very Troubled Child: Therapeutic Practice Innovations in Residential and Educational Settings, edited by Jacquelyn Sanders, PhD, and Barry M. Childress, MD (Vol. 6, No. 4, 1989). *"I find myself wanting to re-read the book-which I recommend for every professional library shelf, especially for directors of programs dealing with the management of residentially located disturbed youth." (Journal of American Association of Psychiatric Administrators)*

The New Board: Changing Issues, Roles and Relationships

Nadia Ehrlich Finkelstein, MS, ACSW
Raymond Schimmer, MAT
Editors

The New Board: Changing Issues, Roles and Relationships has been co-published simultaneously as *Residential Treatment for Children & Youth*, Volume 16, Number 4 1999.

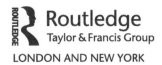

Routledge
Taylor & Francis Group

LONDON AND NEW YORK

The New Board: Changing Issues, Roles and Relationships has been co-published simultaneously as *Residential Treatment for Children & Youth*, Volume 16, Number 4 1999.

First published 1999 by
The Haworth Press, Inc.

Published 2014 by Routledge
2 Park Square, Milton Park, Abingdon, Oxfordshire OX14 4RN
711 Third Avenue, New York, NY 10017

Routledge is an imprint of the Taylor and Francis Group, an informa business

Cover design by Thomas J. Mayshock Jr.

Library of Congress Cataloging-in-Publication Data

The new board : changing issues, roles and relationships / Nadia Ehrlich Finkelstein, Raymond Schimmer, editors.
     p. cm.
    "Co-published simultaneously as Residential treatment for children & youth, volume 16, number 4 1999."
    Includes bibliographical references and index.
    ISBN 978-0-7890-0834-3 (alk. paper)
    1. Child welfare boards–United States. 2. Children–Institutional care–United States. 3. Social work administration–United States. 4. Non-profit organizations–United States. I. Finkelstein, Nadia Ehrlich. II. Schimmer, Raymond.
HV741.N395 1999
362.7'0973–dc21   99-049963

ISBN 978-0-7890-0834-3 (hbk)
ISBN 978-1-138-01229-5 (pbk)

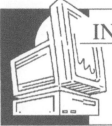

INDEXING & ABSTRACTING

Contributions to this publication are selectively indexed or abstracted in print, electronic, online, or CD-ROM version(s) of the reference tools and information services listed below. This list is current as of the copyright date of this publication. See the end of this section for additional notes.

- *Applied Social Sciences Index & Abstracts (ASSIA) (Online: ASSI via Data-Star) (CDRom: ASSIA Plus)*

- *BUBL Information Service, an Internet-based Information Service for the UK higher education community*

- *Cambridge Scientific Abstracts*

- *Child Development Abstracts & Bibliography*

- *CNPIEC Reference Guide: Chinese National Directory of Foreign Periodicals*

- *Criminal Justice Abstracts*

- *Exceptional Child Education Resources (ECER) (CD/ROM from SilverPlatter and hard copy)*

- *Family Studies Database (online and CD/ROM)*

- *IBZ International Bibliography of Periodical Literature*

- *Index to Periodical Articles Related to Law*

- *International Bulletin of Bibliography on Education*

- *Mental Health Abstracts (online through DIALOG)*

- *National Clearinghouse on Child Abuse & Neglect*

- *National Criminal Justice Reference Service*

- *Psychological Abstracts (PsycINFO)*

- *Sage Family Studies Abstracts (SFSA)*

(continued)

- *Social Planning/Policy & Development Abstracts (SOPODA)*

- *Social Work Abstracts*

- *Sociological Abstracts (SA)*

- *Sociology of Education Abstracts*

- *Special Educational Needs Abstracts*

- *Violence and Abuse Abstracts: A Review of Current Literature on Interpersonal Violence (VAA)*

Special Bibliographic Notes related to special journal issues
(separates) and indexing/abstracting:

- indexing/abstracting services in this list will also cover material in any "separate" that is co-published simultaneously with Haworth's special thematic journal issue or DocuSerial. Indexing/abstracting usually covers material at the article/chapter level.

- monographic co-editions are intended for either non-subscribers or libraries which intend to purchase a second copy for their circulating collections.

- monographic co-editions are reported to all jobbers/wholesalers/approval plans. The source journal is listed as the "series" to assist the prevention of duplicate purchasing in the same manner utilized for books-in-series.

- to facilitate user/access services all indexing/abstracting services are encouraged to utilize the co-indexing entry note indicated at the bottom of the first page of each article/chapter/contribution.

- this is intended to assist a library user of any reference tool (whether print, electronic, online, or CD-ROM) to locate the monographic version if the library has purchased this version but not a subscription to the source journal.

- individual articles/chapters in any Haworth publication are also available through the Haworth Document Delivery Service (HDDS).

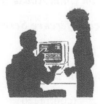

The New Board:
Changing Issues, Roles
and Relationships

CONTENTS

ABOUT THE EDITORS

Nadia Ehrlich Finkelstein, MS, ACSW, is a Child and Family Services Management Specialist. Well known for her contribution to family participation in residential treatment, she has trained and consulted nationally and published extensively in areas addressing permanency needs for children. Her thinking is summarized in *Children and Youth in Limbo, A Search for Connections* (1991). Her forty-five year career in the non-profit child/family sector ranges from direct practice to Associate Executive Director of Parsons Child and Family Center. Ms. Finkelstein holds an MS degree from the Columbia University School of Social Work, is a Life Fellow of the American Association of Children's Residential Centers, an Honorary Life Director of the Board of Directors of Parsons Child and Family Center, a member of the Editorial Board of *Residential Treatment for Children & Youth*, and a member of the National Advisory Board of the Carolina's Project of the Walker Trieschman Center.

Raymond Schimmer, MAT, is Executive Director of Parsons Child and Family Center in Albany, New York. Mr. Schimmer is a graduate of Hunter College and Harvard University School of Education, and has worked in the fields of special education and child welfare for thirty years. He directed Parsons' residential programs for nine years before becoming the Center's Assistant Executive Director in 1992, and is currently a member of the Child Welfare League of America's Residential Care Advisory Board.

ABOUT THE CONTRIBUTORS

Sheldon R. Gelman, PhD, is Professor and Dorothy and David I. Schachne Dean at the Wurzweiler School of Social Work of Yeshiva University in New York. Formerly a professor and director of the social work program at The Pennsylvania State University, he earned his bachelor's degree in psychology and his master's degree in social group work at the University of Pittsburgh. He received his PhD in Welfare Planning from the Heller School of Brandeis University, and his MSL (Master of Studies in Law) from Yale University Law School. Dr. Gelman has published numerous articles dealing with the impact of legislation and policies on the delivery of social services.

Margaret Gibelman, DSW, is Professor and Director of the Doctoral Program at the Wurzweiler School of Social Work of Yeshiva University in New York. She teaches in the areas of social welfare policy, management, and child welfare. She has also taught at Rutgers University and The Catholic University of America. Dr. Gibelman is a frequent contributor to scholarly journals on nonprofit management, privatization, professional education, women's issues, and service delivery systems.

David Kirk, DMin, joined Children's Home & Aid Society of Illinois five years ago as its President and Chief Executive Officer. Under his leadership, this 114 year old statewide child welfare and family service agency has enhanced its governance and service delivery structures through comprehensive strategic planning and board recruitment. Prior to joining the organization, Dr. Kirk served as the President and CEO of ChildServ, a child welfare agency. Dr. Kirk is recognized nationally for his contributions to the field. He serves on the boards of the National Association of Homes & Services for Children and the Child Care Association of Illinois. His other professional affiliations include committee positions with the Child Welfare League of America and the Council on Accreditation of Services for Families and Children, Inc. Dr. Kirk received his undergraduate degree from Marshall University, and graduate degrees from Duke University and Vanderbilt University.

David S. Liederman, MEd, MSW, is President and CEO of the Council on Accreditation of Services for Families and Children, Inc. He was formerly Executive Director of the Child Welfare League of America (CWLA) from 1984-1999. In that role, he has served as the League's national spokesperson, and has promoted the welfare of children and families tirelessly. His professional career has also included youth work in public housing projects, two terms as a Massachusetts State Legislator, and a term as Chief of Staff under

Governor Michael Dukakis. Mr. Liederman earned a Master's of Education at Springfield College and a Master's of Social Work at the University of Pittsburgh. He has served on the faculties of Yeshiva University, the City University of New York, and Boston University.

Judy T. Lindsey, MS, CFRE, is Vice President of Development for Children's Home & Aid Society of Illinois. During her four-year tenure, she has expanded the organization's centralized development operation into a statewide function. Prior to joining Children's Home & Aid Society, Ms. Lindsey was a principal with a development consulting firm, and held clinical and administrative positions with several not-for-profit organizations, including the Assistant Superintendent's post at the Illinois Center for Rehabilitation and Education, a children's residential facility. Ms. Lindsey holds a graduate degree from the University of Wisconsin-Madison, an undergraduate degree from Bradley University, and a post-graduate certificate in rehabilitation administration from DePaul University. As a speaker, Ms. Lindsey has presented at local, regional, and national conferences of the National Society of Fund Raising Executives. She is a past board member of Chicago Cares and Blacks in Development, and serves on the Volunteer Leadership Development Committee of United Way/ Crusade of Mercy in Chicago.

Mildred B. Shapiro, MA, is a health economist and consultant in health and long term care. She is Adjunct Professor of health economics at Union College, Graduate Management Institute, and at the University at Albany School of Public Health. Formerly, she was Associate Commissioner of the New York State Medicaid Program in the New York State Department of Social Services, following a term as Commissioner with the New York State Commission on Quality of Care for the Mentally Disabled. She received a Master of Arts degree in economics from the New School for Social Research.

Elizabeth Skidmore is Associate Director of the National Center for Consultation and Professional Development of the Child Welfare League of America. Ms. Skidmore spent many years as a child welfare administrator in New England, serving as executive director in organizations that provided both residential and community-based care. She has also been Director of Youth Services in Italy for the United States Air Force. Ms. Skidmore's recent research and consultation have focused on board development, strategic planning, and agency organization.

L. D. Williams, MSW, ACSW, was President/CEO of Family & Children's Center, Inc., Mishawaka, Indiana. Family & Children's Center is the corporate parent of six nonprofit 501 C 3 agencies dedicated to providing human services to its clients in the most effective, professional, and economic way. L. D. Williams passed away before publication of this volume.

Foreword

Why this special volume and why now?

In this rapidly changing, globally shrinking world, those of us in the nonprofit Child/Family sector are experiencing many concerns. Although none of these concerns are new or surprising, they seem to be coming to a head: simply defined, the problem is one of survival.

Services to deeply troubled children and their families must be responsive to the social and economic fabric within which these services are provided. A long tradition of committed quality service is no longer sufficient. Market forces have become a fact of life for the nonprofit. Regardless of the quality of their product, failure to respond to this reality will force the nonprofit agency into financial jeopardy.

In one sense, the problems of the nonprofit are even more complicated than those of the for-profit company. The community's charge to our organizations presumes financial integrity but does not stop there. Survival hinges on the ability to fulfill the organization's mission to provide quality services to increasingly more difficult human problems at a time when resources are rapidly shrinking in an economy that, at least at the time of this writing, is doing rather well. These are not issues that professionals can solve alone. The most dedicated competent CEO, chief child psychiatrist, social worker, teacher, and child care worker remain helpless unless the board of directors is so educated and positioned that it can respond rapidly and efficiently in this ever-changing, challenging environment.

For many years, the typical nonprofit organization was overseen by a stable group of board members with a history of long dedicated tenure. The decision pace was slow moving and risk averse. This

[Haworth co-indexing entry note]: "Foreword." Nadia Ehrlich Finkelstein, and Raymond Schimmer. Co-published simultaneously in *Residential Treatment for Children & Youth* (The Haworth Press, Inc.) Vol. 16, No. 4, 1999, pp. xix-xxii; and: *The New Board: Changing Issues, Roles and Relationships* (ed: Nadia Ehrlich Finkelstein, and Raymond Schimmer) The Haworth Press, Inc., 1999, pp. xiii-xvi. Single or multiple copies of this article are available for a fee from The Haworth Document Delivery Service [1-800-342-9678, 9:00 a.m. - 5:00 p.m. (EST). E-mail address: getinfo@haworthpressinc.com].

xiii

culture minimized pressure on the board to move quickly and aggressively. For some board members, this style seemed acceptable. Yet increasingly to others, the "rubber-stamping" of professional activities became ever more frustrating.

As these traditional board members began to retire in significant numbers, board recruitment and composition has become an issue for many organizations. In contrast to the for-profit board member, for whom there are many financial rewards to balance a fast-moving, high-risk pace, the nonprofit board member serves as a volunteer. There, of course, is no financial remuneration of any kind. Yet, as the population requiring service becomes more and more troubled, the assumption of risk increases.

Fortunately, there is a new emergent group of directors, ready to share their experience and competence from the business and professional world, knowing that they are contributing to their communities. They bring the pace of the for-profit world to the board table; business as usual is no longer possible. Given the changing economic and political environment, these board members bring expertise in finance, managed care, organizational management; they are also savvy with mergers and acquisitions. Depending on the size of the nonprofit organization, this experience may be either weak or entirely lacking at the professional level. Furthermore, given the cultural diversity of the community seeking services, boards need adequate client and community representation to assure that limited resources are allocated where they are most effective and most needed.

In this new and different environment, a five-year strategic planning process has become obsolete. The board needs rapid continuing training and education so that it can make policy decisions affecting program planning and direction in a timely, responsive manner. The way a board needs to function requires organizational and operational models that are different from those models which have worked in the past.

We have carefully chosen a group of topics and contributors with direct and current organizational experience. The contributors have generously given of their time and expertise to share their understanding of some key critical issues facing the nonprofit sector. We are keenly aware that we have not begun to cover many relevant issues; however, we are pleased to present the following authors and their papers:

Elizabeth Skidmore, in her paper, "Board Leadership 2000–Critical Roles for the New Century," explores the changing role of a nonprofit agency's board of directors in areas of leadership, planning, strategic affiliations, community development and advocacy.

Professor Margaret Gibelman and Dean Sheldon R. Gelman share a wealth of knowledge in their paper, "Safeguarding the Nonprofit Agency: The Role of the Board of Directors in Risk Management." They speak to the oversight and accountability responsibilities of nonprofit boards, given the scrutiny agencies are experiencing by funding and regulatory bodies.

Dr. David Kirk and Judy T. Lindsey, in "The Changing Role of Trustees in Fund Raising for Residential Treatment Centers," discuss their ideas on effective involvement of trustees in planning and program policy as these relate to the board's role in fund raising. Their comments are the result of a two-year journey into these issues in their agency.

Mildred B. Shapiro, in her paper, "Boards of Directors and Agencies Adapting to Managed Care," brings her vast body of knowledge and experience to this critical new issue for the nonprofit organization. She speaks to both promise and risk in this environment, as well as to critical training issues for directors as they seek to take advantage of these new funding streams on behalf of their agencies.

L. D. Williams addresses "Alternative Board Structures to Accommodate New Demands." He speaks from the perspective of nonprofit management experience, offers several models but describes a very innovative, challenging approach adopted by his own agency.

Nadia Ehrlich Finkelstein and Raymond Schimmer, in "The Board Change Process: One Agency's Experience," describe how one board of directors chose to effect change to assume the challenges and opportunities of this new era.

In addition to thanking our contributors for sharing their knowledge, we would like to thank David S. Liederman, President and CEO of the Council on Accreditation of Services for Families and Children, Inc., formerly Executive Director of the Child Welfare League of America, for writing the Preface to this collection, and Dr. Gordon Northrup, Editor of *Residential Treatment for Children & Youth*, for giving us the opportunity to share the topics of this volume with you. His patience, guidance and confidence in us has been invaluable. We owe our appreciation to the Board of Directors of Parsons Child and

Family Center for providing us with an environment supportive of this endeavor; to Thomas Luzzi, Associate Executive Director of Parsons Child and Family Center, for generously sharing his ideas about critical issues facing the nonprofit board of the future; to Kathryn M. Neuhart, Computer Training and Support Specialist, Parsons Child and Family Center, for technical support; and to Elizabeth A. Waite, Executive Assistant, Parsons Child and Family Center, for her patience, good humor and, above all, technical skill in putting this volume together.

And lastly, we want to emphasize that the thoughts and ideas presented here are those of the individual contributors exclusively, which has allowed for a rich variety of styles and approaches.

Nadia Ehrlich Finkelstein, MS, ACSW
Raymond Schimmer, MAT

Preface:
Today's Nonprofit Board–
A National Perspective

The nonprofit board has been compared to a rudder, keeping an organization's ship on course through the stormy seas of change. But unlike a rudder, which is a solid board or a single piece of metal, an agency board of directors is a complex and shifting group of individuals that interacts with other individuals to steer a complex and shifting organization. After 14 years with my hand on the tiller at CWLA, I have learned a few things about boards, some of which might apply to the boards of treatment centers. The first thing is that they're never simple.

Human beings never have been simple, even as individuals, and much less in the aggregate. But in the old days, most of our organizations were steered by collections of prosperous, middle-aged Caucasians whose views of the world were happily homogeneous. The majority of the community–and the vast majority of the people the agency served–never got near the table. Life was simpler in the old days. And we wouldn't want to go back there even if we could.

Today's best agency boards reflect the diverse backgrounds and perspectives of the communities they represent and the people they serve. Real, substantial diversity–not just tokenism–is absolutely better for all concerned. But it does not always make for smooth sailing.

Change is the constant of our time. Increasing diversity is just one of its aspects. Agencies have to be flexible and agile: faithful to the maps that chart their mission, but able to tack with the wind and even

[Haworth co-indexing entry note]: "Preface: Today's Nonprofit Board–A National Perspective." David S. Liederman. Co-published simultaneously in *Residential Treatment for Children & Youth* (The Haworth Press, Inc.) Vol. 16, No. 4, 1999, pp. xxiii-xxv; and: *The New Board: Changing Issues, Roles and Relationships* (ed: Nadia Ehrlich Finkelstein, and Raymond Schimmer) The Haworth Press, Inc., 1999, pp. xvii-xix. Single or multiple copies of this article are available for a fee from The Haworth Document Delivery Service [1-800-342-9678, 9:00 a.m. - 5:00 p.m. (EST). E-mail address: getinfo@haworthpressinc.com].

xvii

revise the map when the mission shifts. This is hard work. It calls for a fully engaged, committed board and a clear definition of the respective roles of board members, staff members, and administrators.

Fortunately, even in today's stormy climate of rapidly accelerating change, some facts about the role of the board remain the same. Our increasingly diverse boards of directors bring a wider variety of what effective boards have always brought: resources, connections, and expertise. Because organizations naturally tend to focus inward, one major function of your board is to turn you outward: to direct your attention to the outside world, to remind you of its standards, and to connect you with its riches. You need this outward direction and those outside resources more today than ever before.

If you're the executive director, you were hired for your leadership ability, your skill in management, and your commitment to the mission. You hired your staff for their professional backgrounds in child welfare, clinical work, personnel, finance, records management, and other areas of specific expertise. What you need from your board is outside expertise that complements all this–in business, market research, public relations, etc.–and access to vital resources. Today, as always, board members must be committed to your mission, but the last thing you want is a board composed exclusively of social workers or clinicians. Aside from being redundant, that would hardly represent the community in its diversity. Be hard-nosed about this! If board members aren't contributing needed knowledge or other resources, they're just taking up space.

On the other hand, since they're volunteers, you owe them something too. Being a board member is a demanding job. It's up to you to see that it's not a thankless one. Annual dinners and tokens of appreciation are fine, but don't forget the basics. Give them the information they need to do their job well, beginning with an orientation thorough enough to help prospective board members make an informed decision. Then keep educating them, while you give them plenty of opportunities to educate you.

If your board members carry enough weight in the community to bring significant resources to the table, they're busy people. Don't waste their time with unnecessary or poorly managed meetings. I think most local boards meet too often, taking up too much of the board members' time and too much staff time. Six meetings a year is probably the maximum. Put some of the time you save on meetings into planning the agenda, so sessions don't bog down in trivia or rehashing what has already happened. The board's task is to develop large-scale policy, the kind that creates results in the real world. That's leadership. The agency board, like the agency as a whole, needs to be proactive and forward looking.

You can expect people to snooze, or simply to stay away, if the board is so large as to be unwieldy or if you haven't created a climate where it's safe to disagree. Every mariner knows that a good storm clears the air. You need ground rules for disagreement, but if your board is as diverse as it ought to be, you can expect healthy differences of opinion. Who wants to attend a boring meeting?

Board gurus John and Miriam Carver point out that inclusiveness isn't the only way to increase diversity. Since a large board isn't agile, and a board small enough to be efficient can never represent every stakeholder group in the community, the board's orientation and continuing education should include opportunities for face to face contact with the people your agency serves. This will introduce still other points of view and more kinds of conflict, but that's part of the hard work they signed on to do. You don't want cheap consensus; you want the kind of common ground that comes from exploring many angles. Embrace diversity every way you can, hear all sides, but then press on to a responsible decision that gives the organization a unified direction—that keeps it on course. Ideally, that course will include a balance between respect for tradition and openness to change. As your board helps you steer into the future, it must also safeguard your agency's past.

I hope this presentation and the many points of view it introduces will help administrators of treatment agencies develop mutually enriching relationships with their boards, for the sake of the children and families they serve. Bon voyage!

David S. Liederman, MEd, MSW
President and CEO
Council on Accreditation of Services
for Families and Children, Inc.,
formerly Executive Director
of the Child Welfare League of America

Board Leadership 2000–
Critical Roles for the New Century

Elizabeth Skidmore

SUMMARY. In the turbulent and ever-changing human services arena, the meaningful involvement of an active, diverse and committed board of directors may be the key to survival for many nonprofit organizations. This article explores the changing role of a nonprofit agency's board of directors in areas of leadership, planning, strategic affiliations, community development and advocacy. Specific tools and strategies to improve board effectiveness and development to meet the increased demands of a competitive marketplace are recommended. *[Article copies available for a fee from The Haworth Document Delivery Service: 1-800-342-9678. E-mail address: getinfo@haworthpressinc.com <Website: http://www.haworthpressinc.com>]*

KEYWORDS. Nonprofits, boards, management, leadership, strategic planning

ARE NONPROFIT BOARDS IRRELEVANT?

Let there be no doubt: the dramatic political and social changes of the last ten years have created a new set of challenges for most human services agencies. Managed Care, performance based contracting, privatization, shrinking public resources, and the emphasis on quality assurance and outcomes have forced many nonprofits to reexamine the conventional strategies traditionally associated with operating a

---

[Haworth co-indexing entry note]: "Board Leadership 2000–Critical Roles for the New Century." Skidmore, Elizabeth. Co-published simultaneously in *Residential Treatment for Children & Youth* (The Haworth Press, Inc.) Vol. 16, No. 4, 1999, pp. 1-18; and: *The New Board: Changing Issues, Roles and Relationships* (ed: Nadia Ehrlich Finkelstein, and Raymond Schimmer) The Haworth Press, Inc., 1999, pp. 1-18. Single or multiple copies of this article are available for a fee from The Haworth Document Delivery Service [1-800-342-9678, 9:00 a.m. - 5:00 p.m. (EST). E-mail address: getinfo@haworthpressinc.com].

1

nonprofit organization. Yet, while many CEOs have adapted to meet the demands of this new competitive environment, most boards of directors are still operating with the misguided notion of business as usual (Chait, Taylor, 1989).

In the turbulent and ever-changing human services arena, the meaningful involvement of an active, diverse and committed board of directors may be the key to survival for many nonprofit organizations. As J. Gregory Dees points out in his article, "Enterprising Nonprofits,"

> Many nonprofits simply do not have the business-specific skills, managerial capacity, and credibility to succeed in commercial markets. And building new organizational capabilities can be costly and difficult. (Dees, 1998, p. 59)

Nonprofit boards often include their communities' finest business leaders, entrepreneurs, administrators and community activists. These individuals bring a wealth of experience, knowledge and problem-solving skills to their positions as board leaders and are extremely adept at successfully negotiating in the competitive marketplace. Creating effective business strategies, recruiting talented staff, sales, marketing, management information technology and managed care expertise, etc., are just a few of the additional skills that board leaders may offer a nonprofit organization, skills critically important in the current environment.

Unfortunately, many board members are never given the chance to contribute their respective talents to the organizations they've pledged to serve. As Richard P. Chait and Barbara Taylor (1989) underscore in their article, "Charting the Territory of Nonprofit Boards," board members get "bogged down in operating details, matters that are best left to staff, while ignoring the very issues that could determine the enterprise's success or failure." Why, then, do CEOs relegate the most talented and able individuals associated with their organization to the tasks which require few skills: approving minutes, policies and committee reports? Ultimately, even the most dedicated professionals and community leaders become frustrated or bored with their roles as head nodders and stop showing up for meetings or resign (Taylor, Chait, Holland, 1996).

For many years, the Child Welfare League of America's Center for Consultation and Professional Development has worked extensively with CEOs and board members to redirect the time, talents and commitment of board volunteers toward work that has a greater impact on their organization. Many board members are no longer satisfied to simply approve minutes and make an annual donation. As one board member recently stated, "I'm too busy to sit around simply agreeing with the CEO's agenda; I want to make a meaningful contribution to the organization and to furthering its mission." In turn, CEOs often struggle with trying to maintain a balance between keeping board members out of operations while keeping them sufficiently engaged in governance. Intent in their effort to keep board members in line, some CEOs fail to harness the talents of individuals who may be in the best position to ultimately ensure the organization's (and their) success.

Even the most experienced CEOs often have difficulty ensuring that their board members realize the value of their contributions. In situations where board volunteers view their CEO's leadership as effective and competent, they often believe that their help isn't really needed, or at times, appreciated. Unfamiliar with the intricacies of public funding, social service programming, etc., some board members are hesitant to question the skills and experience most nonprofit CEOs have attained during their professional lifetimes. These perceptions often result in poor attendance, boring discussions, and show and tell meetings "hosted" by the CEO. Determining how best to actively engage board members in work that is interesting, has meaning and makes a significant difference to the future of the organization, therefore, is an important challenge for CEOs and board leaders alike. Research from the University of Southern California's Marshall School for Effective Organizations indicates that boards need "knowledge, information, power, motivation and time" to perform their job efficiently (Conger, Finegold, Lawlor, 1998). Achieving this goal, therefore, must be primary to a nonprofit organization's board development strategy. Empowering board members to assume new and different responsibilities in order to become effective, strategic and visionary leaders, however, is even more important.

The question becomes, what are the new responsibilities of board members in the current environment? What skills will board leaders need in the future to secure the viability of their organization's mission *and* business? How can CEOs forge partnerships with their board leaders that strengthen and enhance an agency's value to its customers and community? Finally, what structures and tools can boards and CEOs employ to direct, clarify and simplify their work?

FOCUSING ON MISSION

During a workshop offered for board members by the Child Welfare League of America, the facilitator asked a group of experienced board leaders from across the country, "What is the primary responsibility of a board member in a child welfare organization?" More than twenty different answers, ranging from fund development to policy approval, were given in response to this question. Participants in the workshop also disagreed regarding the level and type of involvement board leaders should assume in their nonprofit organizations. If this small sample is representative of most nonprofit boards, confusion reigns regarding the focus of board leadership.

Board leaders in for-profit companies understand that the bottom line is ensuring that the corporation makes a profit (Lesser, 1991). Other board responsibilities and tasks are evaluated and understood in terms of how earnings are generated and/or impacted. The for-profit organization's mission exists primarily to generate profits (see Figure 1). At Ford Motor Company, for example, their well-marketed mission statement promotes, "Quality is job one." Yet Ford's commitment to their mission of quality is directly tied to their belief that quality impacts profits.

In contrast, the bottom line in nonprofit organizations is mission. Nonprofit organizations exist because of their mission. Financial resources are developed for the sole purpose of furthering the organization's mission. As evidenced in Figure 1, the nonprofit board member's primary responsibility, therefore, is ensuring that their nonprofit organization promotes, protects and delivers its mission in the same manner a for-profit corporation delivers profits to its shareholders.

According to management expert Peter Drucker (1991), focusing

FIGURE 1

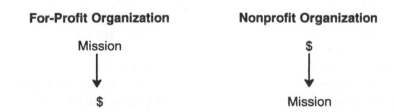

on mission means that board members have an obligation to ensure that the mission achieves results. Indeed, mission results are central to a nonprofit's survival in the future. Authors Eugene Fram and Robert Pierce (1992) agree. As they state in their management guide for boards and executives, "The High Performance Nonprofit," "If non-profit organizations are to thrive, the executive director and board must always be attuned to productivity and performance issues" (Fram, Pierce, p. 4).

Unfortunately, however, few boards make time to discuss either mission or results during their monthly or quarterly meetings. Tradition or history dictates the configuration of agendas, meetings and committees of many nonprofits, even when these models no longer serve a definitive purpose. Boards of directors intent on providing effective leadership must defy "the conventions that have regulated board behavior in the past" (Taylor et al., 1996, p. 36). Board leaders need to reassess, reorganize and reinvigorate board structures to ensure that their organization achieves its mission, delivers results and is strategically positioned for the future. Committees, task forces and meetings need to be focused on what matters, "the crucial, do or die issues central to the institution's success" (Taylor et al., 1996, p. 36).

BOARD MEMBERS AS STRATEGISTS

In a recent article featured in *Harvard Business Review,* "The New Work of the Nonprofit Board," authors Barbara Taylor, Richard Chait and Thomas Holland emphasize:

> A board's contribution is meant to be strategic, the joint product of talented people brought together to apply their knowledge and experience to meet the major challenges facing the institution. (1996, p. 36)

Unfortunately, many boards believe their responsibility to the organization's strategic development begins and ends with the creation of a five-year strategic plan. These documents typically gather dust in the CEO's file cabinet, only to be rediscovered during the next strategic planning cycle.

In contrast, savvy business leaders have long understood that the traditional method of strategic planning isn't effective in a rapidly changing, competitive marketplace. Many for-profit companies have reinvented their strategic planning approach to become a more dynamic and fluid process "because," argues Henry Mintzberg (1994), author and former president of the Strategic Management Society, "strategic development is about change and one can never know when or how environments will change." In many companies across America, business leaders plan strategy daily, if not hourly. A primary focus of for-profit board meetings is strategic development. Yet, although business leaders have recognized the critical importance of the shift to a revitalized strategic planning process in their own industry, they often fail to understand its value to the nonprofit world. If board leaders are to adequately prepare their nonprofit for the twenty-first century, they must view their role in strategy development differently.

During a fall summit of seventy board leaders from throughout New England hosted by the Child Welfare League of America, several board members spoke candidly about the new challenges facing their organizations. They articulated an understanding of the current human services environment, identified issues critical to their organization's strategic development and spoke passionately about vision. Other board members expressed surprise regarding the breadth of knowledge displayed by their board colleagues. "How do you know so much about child welfare?" asked one board leader. "I've been on my board seven years and don't even know what I don't know."

Crucial to all effective strategic planning processes is providing decision makers with information about an industry's trends and environment. One of a CEO's primary responsibilities, therefore, must be ensuring that his/her board of directors has the knowledge required to understand the compelling issues impacting the organization so that they may be full partners in the strategic planning process. A recent article on board leadership points out:

> The litmus test of the chief executive's leadership is not the ability to solve problems alone but the capacity to articulate key questions and guide a collaborative effort to formulate answers. (Taylor et al., p. 37)

If board leaders are sufficiently informed regarding the current and future trends facing their nonprofit organizations, they will quickly grasp the need for ongoing, dynamic strategic planning efforts and development by board membership. As one board president recently said, "I finally understand that my job here (as board president) is much the same as my job at work: developing strategy, ensuring results, reducing risks."

Given the importance ongoing strategic planning now signifies to nonprofits, CEOs must ensure that a majority of their board members are strategic thinkers. "The combined knowledge and experience of the board members absolutely must match the strategic demands of the organization" (Conger et al., p. 140). "Our board doesn't just develop our strategy," states Ted Lewis, CEO of The Children's Center in Detroit, Michigan, "they're part of it." While many CEOs have downsized their board membership over the last ten years, the Children's Center board boasts more than sixty-three board members with another fifty in subcommittees. Some of Detroit's most highly regarded managed care professionals make up the Children's Center managed care subcommittee. Area technology experts plan and evaluate to meet the agency's management information needs, and the real estate developers and professionals have assisted Mr. Lewis with developing a sound real estate strategy.

Nonprofit organizations that include board members as part of a comprehensive "strategic resource" package will benefit tremendously from the skills and talents these volunteers bring to the organization. As Michael Annison (1993) states in his book *Managing the Whirlwind*:

> Strategic Resources are those resources we need to be successful. . . . Now the human mind has become the transforming resource. . . . The knowledge and skills that got us to where we are were necessary, but are not adequate for future success. During periods of stability, we can apply what we have learned in the past to the present and future. During periods of change, we need to keep on learning.

DEVELOPING A STRATEGIC ADVANTAGE THROUGH BOARD COMPOSITION

Nonprofit leaders positioning their organizations for the future must include the skill sets and experience of their board membership as part of their strategic "tool kit." Annually, the board/CEO team should draft a list of the organization's strategic priorities for the coming year

(Conger et al., 1998). Current board members should complete a board matrix (see Appendix A), which assesses the skills of current board membership, diversity and geographic representation. The nominating or board development committee then compares this list against the strategic priorities of the organization to determine what board skills/ experience might be needed in the coming year. If, for example, the CEO and board has determined that their organization should create a planned giving program, build a new facility or invest heavily in technology, the board might pursue a contractor or architect, estate lawyer, planned giving professional and/or management information specialist. In this way, the board's expertise matches the strategic priorities of the organization (Taylor et al., 1996). In addition, "The resulting exchange will be a learning experience for both parties" (Dees, 1998).

This approach does not discount, however, the importance of re-cruiting and retaining board members that bring other resources to the organization. Potential donors, board members with community connections, clients, worker bees, etc., also contribute to the current and future viability of nonprofit boards. Focusing on "the constellation, not the stars" (Taylor et al. 1996) is the most important goal to attain when establishing an effective, strategic and collaborative board of directors.

Another important contribution board leaders bring to a nonprofit organization is diversity of thought, experience and education. In their highly regarded book, *Competing for the Future* (1994), authors Gary Hamel and C. K. Prahalad emphasize the critical importance of avoiding "corporate genetics" in an organization's strategic planning and decision making processes. Corporate genetics refers to the belief that organizational vision is often limited and narrowly focused when strategy is developed by leaders who share the educational background, culture, work experience, politics, value system, etc. Hamel and Prahalad point out:

> These beliefs are, at least in part, the product of a particular industry environment. When that environment changes rapidly and radically, those beliefs may become a threat to survival. (p. 53)

Therefore, if engaged effectively, board membership will provide an opportunity for a nonprofit organization to think, plan and grow beyond the boundaries of its industry and its staff leadership. Few

CEOs who have grown up in the child welfare profession have direct experience or educational background to deal with the realities of a competitive, open market place alone. Faced with competition from managed care companies, highly capitalized for-profit businesses and other nonprofits, CEOs must partner with their board leadership to maximize their collective talents, knowledge and experience as part of a comprehensive strategic planning approach.

THE ROLE OF THE NONPROFIT BOARD IN DEVELOPING STRATEGIC AFFILIATIONS AND MERGERS

A valuable component of any strategic planning process in the current environment is the organization's approach to strategic affiliations. Board members must play a critical role in the brokering and development of strategic relationships with other organizations. As the National Center for Nonprofit Boards points out in its handbook, *Nonprofit Mergers: The Board's Responsibility to Consider the Unthinkable* (1994), "It (mergers) offers one of the clearest calls for board leadership and the strongest appeals to board responsibility that a nonprofit board is likely to face." Driven by economic, political and competitive market concerns, the number of nonprofit organizations that have merged, pursued joint ventures and networks, or been acquired has grown significantly over the past several years (LaPiana, 1997). Providing effective leadership before, during and after an organization develops either a formal or informal strategic affiliation is critical to the healthy formation and maintenance of these relationships.

As a first step, the Board and CEO should determine whether or not strategic affiliations are a necessary component of the broader organizational strategy. CEOs and board members experienced in the art of developing these types of relationships are quick to point out that collaborations and partnerships often look better on paper than in reality (Ashkenas, 1998). Formal affiliations: mergers, acquisitions, joint ventures, networks, etc., can be expensive and full of risks. Inherent to strategic affiliations between nonprofit child welfare agencies, in particular, are enormous liabilities involving the safety of clients. Board members must assess if the benefits of partnering with other organizations to complement their organization's overall strategy outweigh the potential hazards. In his handbook on *Affiliations, Mergers and Acquisitions* (1996), primary author Craig Savage states:

> Once the strategy has been developed, prior to proceeding with negotiation, the organization's leadership must articulate what it expects to gain from any affiliation. This is an exercise which requires careful thought. . . .

When an organization has determined that they wish to pursue a formal partnership, the board plays an even more important role. During negotiations between two nonprofits considering a formal affiliation, board members are responsible for ensuring that the vision and mission of their respective organizations are compatible. As Barbara Schenkel, Chairperson of Youth Alternatives in Portland, Maine states,

> As board members, our primary responsibility is to ensure that Youth Alternatives achieves its mission for the benefit of the Maine community. When an organization is considering a strategic affiliation or merger that could alter the focus or integrity of that organization's mission, the board must be involved. Once the board has agreed upon the compatibility of mission, values and goals with a potential partner, the CEO should be responsible for making the relationship operational.

The board's role during negotiations between potential partners, therefore, is first to represent the mission/vision of the organization. Secondly, the board must ensure that the basic values of the organization are protected and/or enhanced through the strategic relationship. Lastly, the board should determine which strategic goals will be achieved through the creation of the proposed partnership. Other board members might be involved with assessing information obtained through the due diligence process; however, many CEOs and board leaders feel this data is best reviewed by lawyers and other professionals hired by the organization who can offer expertise and objectivity.

Once a strategic affiliation has been formalized, the newly identified CEO assumes primary responsibility for ensuring that the two previously autonomous organizations function as a whole (in the case of a merger, acquisition) or achieve joint goals (as in a joint venture or network). However, while CEOs and board leaders typically find the process of identifying partners and negotiating the relationship manageable, most quickly learn that maintaining an alliance is often the greatest challenge. In her book, *Frontiers of Management* (1997), Rosabeth Moss Kantor states:

> Operational and cultural differences emerge after collaboration is under way. They often come as a surprise to those who created the alliance. That failure could reflect blind spots. . . . Mistrust, once introduced, sets off a vicious cycle. It makes success harder to attain, which means someone has to be blamed. . . . (p. 236)

One of the most difficult challenges many nonprofits have faced is managing the relationship after the affiliation has been formalized. This is an area where board leadership and experience can be extremely valuable to a CEO. Many problems unforeseen during affiliation discussions appear as unwelcome surprises once the organizations have joined together. Financial problems, staff relationships and facility issues are just a few of the troubles that often materialize. "If board members are appropriately involved and informed during all phases of the strategic affiliation process," states Gordon Rehnborg, Chairman of the Board of Directors for Child and Family Services of New Hampshire, "then everyone is equally responsible when the rats come out of the closet afterwards."

BOARD LEADERSHIP IN THE COMMUNITY: A CRITICAL ROLE

Pivotal to the development of any organizational strategy in a nonprofit organization is the input of key community stakeholders and customers. The board must retain a role in these public relations efforts for many reasons. First, voluntary board members serve as their community's representatives to the nonprofit organization. As such, they must be able to understand, clearly articulate and respond to the needs of their constituencies as emphasized in the article, "The High Performing Nonprofit" (Fram and Pearse, 1992):

> In building high performance nonprofit organizations, managers and boards should monitor continually their stakeholders, whose

opinions and behaviors affect organizational performance. Such stakeholders include clients or customers and persons in government, business, and other nonprofit groups. In some ways, all will affect a nonprofit's decision making process. These stakeholders can be either powerful allies or skillful enemies. A high performing nonprofit, whether it be a social agency, trade association, arts group, or other type of organization, will do everything possible to maximize positive stakeholder relationships.

Board members should demand that their organization regularly solicit feedback from funders, consumers and community representatives regarding customer service, effectiveness of programs, reputation, funding trends, etc. Once the board receives this information, it should be incorporated into the organization's overall strategy, program development and quality improvement initiatives.

Secondly, board members have an important role as ambassadors of the organization in their community. Board members are effective advocates, cheerleaders and crisis interventionists when necessary and appropriate. Many times, professional staff members are seen as self-serving when they attempt to advance the mission and business of their employing organizations. Board members who receive no tangible benefit from their association with a nonprofit organization are viewed differently and are able to create important inroads with key decision makers and community leaders otherwise unavailable to nonprofit staff.

In particular, a board's active role in the advocacy efforts of their organization ensures that the broader systemic, political and funding issues that so often provide barriers to a nonprofit's ability to achieve their mission are addressed. As Alan Gratch (1980) of the CWLA so persuasively states:

> Board members and social workers alike have recognized that the specific services that an agency provides constitute only one part of the agency's responsibility for children. There is another part of the child welfare agency's responsibility that may, and often does, help many more children than those who receive its direct services, namely, the agency's active participation in efforts affecting programs, legislation, and attitudes that contribute to the prevention of conditions that cause some of the problems of children and parents. A child welfare agency has a duty to work

to ensure that all children–not just those in its caseload–are given proper care.

In keeping with their commitment to the organization's mission, as well as the issues important to children and families in their community, board leaders must accept and promote their responsibilities as child and family advocates. To be effective advocates and catalysts for change, however, board members must be able to communicate knowledgeably regarding key concerns and stakeholder's needs. Additionally, boards must institutionalize their advocacy efforts by creating an advocacy committee and by integrating advocacy strategies into the organization's broader strategic plan. In this way, board leaders can serve as powerful and dynamic advocates on behalf of children and families. Gratch (1980) emphasizes this point:

> As responsible, caring humans, as fiduciaries accountable for the past, present, and future of their respective agencies and the children and families served, as leaders in the community, board members are duty bound to front the attack. (p. 31)

A final rationale for board members to take an active role in establishing a comprehensive public relations strategy in their organization is fund development. As the basis of all successful fund development strategies rests with a nonprofit's ability to engage their community and current/potential supporters around the value of the organization's mission, board members are in an important position to directly impact the financial health of their organization. Board members, not CEOs, have greater influence with corporations, donors, United Ways, foundations, etc. Indeed, many foundations now require a minimum donation from every board member in order for the organization to be considered for a grant. However uncomfortable a board member might be with the fund development process, their involvement with any one donor, business or foundation is often the difference in their nonprofit's financial future.

MAXIMIZING THE RELATIONSHIP
BETWEEN BOARDS AND CEOs

Much of the success of focused and skillful board leadership must be attributed to a strong, capable CEO. A board is responsible for seeing that their organization "has the highest caliber CEO and executive team possible" (Conger, 1998). As nonprofit organizations shift to accommodate the demands of a changing human services environment, many boards must rethink the skills and experience their CEO will need to successfully lead their organization into the future.

Consider the dilemma faced by a board of directors of a medium-sized child welfare agency in Washington, DC. Board members were evenly split regarding two finalists for their CEO position. Both candidates had excellent references, educational backgrounds and experience. One candidate had over twenty years of experience as a practitioner and supervisor of a variety of child welfare programs. The second candidate had never worked in a child welfare organization, yet had extensive experience as a community activist, grant writer, entrepreneur and small business owner. Ultimately, the board of directors selected the second candidate. A year later, the group remains highly satisfied with their decision.

How did the board finally determine which applicant was the best choice? In this scenario, the board revisited the organization's strategic goals and looked at industry trends. Both factors helped board members to see the importance of hiring a CEO who could best negotiate a fast paced and competitive environment–a much different selection than they would probably have made two years ago. James Gelatt (1992) echoes this sentiment in his book, *Managing Nonprofit Organizations in the 21st Century.*

> There are dramatic changes in demographics, in values, in health care and education, in science and technology–all of which will alter irrevocably the way in which successful nonprofit organizations will be structured and managed. The image of the manager of the 1970s or even the 1980s will not fit the manager of the year 2000. While there are some common characteristics of managers in general, it is safe to say that what worked in the nonprofits of 1980 may not work at all in the twenty-first century. (p. viii)

Therefore, if Mr. Gelatt is accurate, board leaders will be challenged not only to hire CEOs with different skills and experience, but they must also ensure that their present CEOs receive the training, support and mentorship they need to move their organization successfully into the future.

Understandably, board leaders are often hesitant to encourage their

CEO to pursue additional training and professional development activities, especially when these same individuals have had a successful track record in the past. CEOs are equally reticent about asking their board for help, believing that they'll be perceived as incompetent. Unfortunately, when boards and CEOs fail to connect regarding the executive abilities needed to operate a nonprofit organization in the present environment and in the future, the CEO may end up on the losing side. Worse yet, the organization, bereft of deliberate, effective and farsighted leadership, might be placed in jeopardy. Therefore, ensuring that the CEO has the capabilities necessary to safeguard the organization's mission and future is clearly an important responsibility of the board of directors. As management expert Rosabeth Moss Kantor (1997) so eloquently states, "Leaders create the future by emphasizing what the company's people must learn, not by reinforcing what they already know."

One way to ameliorate problems with CEO performance is through a comprehensive evaluation. Too often, board leaders invest insufficient time and resources in this important process. As the National Center for NonProfit Boards (Pierson, Mintz, 1995) points out:

> In too many nonprofit organizations across the country, the board seldom—if ever—takes the time to assess the chief executive's performance. In many cases, the assessment is perfunctory and may not produce useful results for the executive or organization. When the executive does receive feedback, it is often during a period of change or stress, hardly a time when effective dialogue can take place.

There are three components to a useful CEO evaluation. First, the CEO must be evaluated based upon his or her achievement of previously established goals. The board of directors and CEO should negotiate these objectives annually, and tie several directly to the broader strategic goals of the organization. Additionally, the board should establish goals which assess a CEO's leadership ability and his/her working relationship with the board. "Best practice companies kept their (objective list) to between five and ten objectives" (Conger et al., 1998).

A second, and sometimes unpopular, phase of a comprehensive CEO evaluation is gathering information from stakeholders, peers, subordinates and supervisors regarding organizational and CEO performance.

Often referred to as a 360-degree assessment, more and more nonprofit organizations are following the lead of their business counterparts to include the input of internal and external sources as part of their CEO evaluation. Using this model, feedback is typically collected through a variety of methods including interviews, focus groups and organizational surveys (Hays Group, 1996). Once assessed, this information is used to help substantiate CEO performance in the organization, in the community, and in the broader human services arena.

Lastly, the CEO must furnish a self-evaluation that provides a summary of performance over the previous year. Not only is a self-evaluation a valuable professional development tool for the CEO, but it can also serve as an excellent foundation for creating the following year's performance objectives.

Combined, these three components of an effective performance appraisal allow board members to assess their CEO based upon feedback received from internal and external sources, measurable objectives and results, and self-evaluation–a comprehensive, substantiated and diverse set of information. Engaged in this type of CEO evaluation, board members can feel confident regarding their CEOs (and organization's) performance. Further, should concerns arise regarding one or two areas of a CEO's competency or skill, boards can easily target resources and remedial efforts on the identified problem area. In turn, CEOs receive honest, supportable feedback regarding their strengths, weaknesses and challenges–information most CEOs welcome. As Sue Krahe, CEO of Our Town in Tucson, Arizona recently stated: "How else can I grow as a leader and as a person if I don't receive honest assessments of my performance?"

Leading a child welfare agency into the year 2000 promises to challenge the most capable boards of directors and the best entrepreneurial and talented CEOs. Too often, responsibility for the leadership and momentum of an organization rests solely with the CEO–a highly complex, risky and difficult job that could be made much easier with a fully engaged board partner. The organizational and industry reform needed for most nonprofits to succeed in the future is directly linked to the ability of board leaders and CEOs to present "multiple perspectives and develop solutions that reflect the group's best thinking." Only in this way can we ensure that child and family service organizations and other nonprofits will survive to serve tomorrow's children, families and communities.

REFERENCES

Annison, Michael (1993). *Managing the Whirlwind*, Colorado, Medical Group Management Association.

Chait, Richard P., Taylor, Barbara (Jan.-Feb. 1998). Charting the Territory of Non-Profit Boards, *Harvard Business Review*, 44-54.

Conger, Jay A., Finegold, David, Lawler III, Edward, E. (Jan.-Feb. 1998). Appraising Boardroom Performance, *Harvard Business Review*, 136-148.

Drucker, Peter, It Profits Us to Strengthen Nonprofits, *Wall Street Journal*, Dec. 1991.

Fenn, Donna (Nov. 1997). Sleeping with the Enemy, *Inc.*, 78-86.

Fram, Eugene H., Pearse, Robert (1992). The High Performance Nonprofit, Families International Inc., 1-11.

Gelatt, James P. (1992). *Managing Nonprofit Organizations in the 21st Century*, Phoenix, Arizona, Oryx Press.

Gratch, Alan S. (1980). *Board Members Are Child Advocates*, Child Welfare League of America, Washington, DC.

Hamel, Gary & Prahalad, C. K. (1994). *Competing for the Future*. Boston, Massachusetts, Harvard Business School Press.

Hays Group, *Workshop Presentation on 360 Degree Assessments*, 1996, New York.

Kantor, Rosabeth Moss (1997). *Frontiers of Management*, Boston, Massachusetts, Harvard Business School Press.

LaPiana, David (1997). Strategic Restructuring: Tools for Survival and Success, *Caring*.

Lesser, Lawrence M. (Dec. 1991). For-Profit Attitude Is Key to Nonprofit Productivity, *Washington Post*.

Mintzberg, Henry (1994). *The Rise and Fall of Strategic Planning*, New York, Free Press.

National Center for Nonprofit Boards (1994). *NonProfit Mergers: The Board's Responsibility to Consider the Unthinkable*, Washington, DC.

Pierson, Jane, Mintz, Joshua (1996). *Assessment of the Chief Executive*, National Center for Non Profit Boards.

Savage, Craig, M. (1996). *Affiliations, Mergers and Acquisitions: Guidelines for Pursuing Corporate Integration for Behavioral Services Providers*, Tallahassee, Florida, National Community Mental Health Council.

Senge, Peter M. (1990). *The Fifth Discipline: The Art and Practice of The Learning Organization*. New York, Currency Doubleday.

Taylor, Barbara, E., Chait, Richard P., Holland, Thomas P. (Sept.-Oct. 1996). The New Work of the Nonprofit Board, *Harvard Business Review*, 36-46.

APPENDIX A: BOARD MATRIX

Representation and Skills										
Diversity Representation										
Age										
Gender										
Race										
Community Representation										
Business										
Education										
Public Sector										
Community Networks etc.										
Church										
Skills										
Personnel										
Marketing										
MIS										
Development										
Managed Care										
Legal										
Planned Giving										
Strategic Planning										
Other Criteria (to be determined)										

Safeguarding the Nonprofit Agency:
The Role of the Board of Directors
in Risk Management

Margaret Gibelman, DSW
Sheldon R. Gelman, PhD

SUMMARY. The board of directors of human service agencies has a pivotal role in overseeing the policies, procedures and operations of the service organization. This article explores the role of boards of directors in safeguarding nonprofit organizations through the management of risk and application of overall good judgment. Safeguarding refers to the oversight and accountability function of boards in relation to how business is conducted. Included are considerations pertaining to protection of consumer interests, assurances of quality services, positive and documented outcomes, and full compliance with laws, regulations, and professional standards pertaining to how nonprofit organizations are expected to operate on behalf of those served. The role of nonprofit boards in risk management is reviewed, with particular reference to the implementation of this role in nonprofit residential treatment settings. Strategies to enhance board functioning in the risk management arena are detailed and recommendations are offered about overall organizational preparation and practices for managing risk. *[Article copies available for a fee from The Haworth Document Delivery Service: 1-800-342-9678. E-mail address: getinfo@haworthpressinc.com <Website: http://www.haworthpressinc.com>]*

KEYWORDS. Nonprofits, boards, risk management, management

[Haworth co-indexing entry note]: "Safeguarding the Nonprofit Agency: The Role of the Board of Directors in Risk Management." Gibelman, Margaret, and Sheldon R. Gelman. Co-published simultaneously in *Residential Treatment for Children & Youth* (The Haworth Press, Inc.) Vol. 16, No. 4, 1999, pp. 19-37; and: *The New Board: Changing Issues, Roles and Relationships* (ed: Nadia Ehrlich Finkelstein, and Raymond Schimmer) The Haworth Press, Inc., 1999, pp. 19-37. Single or multiple copies of this article are available for a fee from The Haworth Document Delivery Service [1-800-342-9678, 9:00 a.m. - 5:00 p.m. (EST). E-mail address: getinfo@haworthpressinc.com].

One of the hallmarks of the past decade is the growing trend to litigate disputes and grievances and the increasing involvement of the courts and state and federal legislatures in how and how well human services are organized, delivered, and evaluated (Trumper, 1989, 1994). The competence of human services professionals has been under scrutiny, and there is an increasing demand for accountability for the process, quality, and outcome of services (Kearns, 1996).

MANAGING RISK

Risk management refers to the policies, procedures, and processes of an organization designed to reduce the chances of liability exposure. Risk management strategies are actualized through the board of directors and its delegates to reduce legal vulnerability (Bryant & Korsak, 1988; Gelman, 1987, 1992; Monagle, 1985). In a proactive manner, risk management implies that the organization manages its business in accord with both sound financial practices and applicable laws, regulations, and professional requirements. The business of the organization is conducted in such a way as to reduce risk through evaluation of potential risks which it may assume and implementation of strategic plans to ensure legal, ethical, and professional accountability (Council on Accreditation, 1997). Managing risk is a prevention-oriented and ongoing activity to improve the quality of services and prevent negative outcomes (Tremper, 1994).

The need to minimize risk is both good practice and an organizational requirement, given the rise in the actual and potential number of complaints against human service agencies and their personnel. The need for practical tools that can help develop and guide good practice based on legal, ethical, and sound business principles is clear. Areas in which human service organizations are increasingly vulnerable include negligence, breach of duty through acts of omission or commission, conflict of interest, confidentiality, privileged communication, informed consent, quality of service, contracts, and "unorthodox" treatment (Antler, 1985; Besharov, 1985; Gelman, 1983, 1995; Joseph, 1989). The range of complaints against human service agencies and/or practitioners include sexual improprieties, incompetence and/or incorrect treatment, breach of confidentiality/privacy, misrepresentation through marketing, breach of duty/failure to warn, abandonment of clients (certainly an increasingly important issue in a managed care environment), defamation/libel/slander, and exerting undue influence (Gelman, 1988, 1989; Roswell, 1988).

REASON FOR CONCERN

Risk management as a practice is within the jurisdiction of the board of directors. Implementation functions may be delegated to staff, but the ultimate responsibility lies within the board. It is in the distinction between oversight and day-to-day operations that role conflicts may occur. Recent media revelations about the wrongdoings of nonprofit organizations suggest that the oversight role of boards in risk management may not be widely understood. Aggregate data on the number of such incidences of boards being "caught" are not available. It is clear, however, that suspicion and disparagement has been cast upon the nonprofit sector in general, the results of which may reverberate in tighter government regulations, donor skepticism, and greater demands upon and expectations of governing boards (Gibelman, Gelman & Pollack, 1997). Consideration of the board's role in risk management is particularly important within the context of escalating demand for the services provided by nonprofits, intense competition for the funds that drive these services, and the growing acknowledgment of the role of voluntary leadership in the success of nonprofit organizations (Axelrod, 1994).

Recent discussions in the literature have heightened our collective awareness of the trouble in which nonprofit boards may find themselves if risk is not appropriately managed. Examples include the United Way of America, National Association for the Advancement of Colored People, Foundation for a New Era Philanthropy, Jewish Community Center of Greater Washington, and Upsala College. (For a comprehensive review of these cases, see Gibelman, Gelman & Pollack, 1997; Gelman, Gibelman, Pollack, & Schnall, 1996; Kearns, 1996.) In all of these instances, appropriate board oversight could have prevented the harm that befell them, their constituencies, and the communities and constituencies they serve. At the very heart of the issue is clarification of the role and functions of boards.

THE ROLE AND FUNCTIONS OF THE BOARD

Laws relating to the incorporation of nonprofit organizations require that a board of directors be created to assume basic responsibility for the operations of the corporation. Agency charters and bylaws, in turn, specify the responsibilities and obligations of boards and their individual members. Whereas boards of public agencies are advisory or administrative and therefore do not have as broad powers or responsibilities, boards of directors or trustees of private or voluntary organizations are charged with the general direction and control of those organizations (Mitton, 1974). Thus, the board is the policy making body of the organization, with a legal duty to ensure that the agency's actions are consistent with its goals and objectives.

Board members share collective responsibility for the fiscal and programmatic aspects of the organization's performance. However ambiguous its role in terms of the day-to-day operations of the organization (depending in part on the organization's size, scope, and stage of development), the board is responsible to funding sources, to the community, to governmental and private regulating bodies, and to consumers of service. Simply put, the buck stops with the board (Gelman, 1995; Gibelman, Gelman, & Pollack, 1997).

Board members thus have a legal and moral obligation to keep themselves fully informed about the agency's operations. In addition to the planning and policy making functions, the board is also responsible for the general direction and control of the agency. Other roles include hiring and evaluating the chief executive officer, facilitating fund raising and access to necessary resources, and representing the organization within the larger community context. Finally, the board is also responsible for evaluating the effectiveness of the agency and its responsiveness to community and constituent needs (Axelrod, 1994; Gelman, 1995). Each of these designated areas of responsibility encompass and include a risk management component.

LEGAL OBLIGATIONS

Nonprofit corporations need volunteer directors who will hold themselves and the corporation to the highest standards of accountability. Board members assume *fiduciary* responsibility—a duty to act for the good of others (Axelrod, 1994). The directors of nonprofit corporations are required to exercise reasonable and ordinary care in the performance of their duties, exhibiting honesty and good faith. They must discharge their duties with the degree of care, skill, and diligence any prudent person would exercise under similar circumstances.

It is the board of directors that, as a group, manages the nonprofit corporation, delegating responsibilities appropriately, but retains ultimate responsibility for the agency's image and performance (Hanson & Marmaduke, 1972). The board of directors is legally and morally accountable to the agency's various constituencies for its actions or inaction. According to Gelman (1983, p. 88), "a board which fails in its function of both determining policy and evaluating achievement in support of those policies is negligent in performing its mandated functions." Should that occur, board members risk not only personal monetary liability, but also their reputations as competent and responsible community leaders (Siciliano & Spiro, 1992). The reputation of the agency is at stake, with potential ramifications for the consumers who are served.

To ensure the well-being of the organization, the board must act prudently and lead the organization by developing and implementing a viable method for reviewing its performance and evaluating achievements and movement toward goal attainment (Anthes, 1985; Leifer & Glomb, 1992). This involves periodically subjecting itself to external and internal risk analysis. These are not one-time responsibilities. Unfortunately, it cannot be assumed that boards remain vigilant in addressing these functions. Six areas in which charges of negligence can involve board members have been identified: failure to manage and supervise the activities of the corporation, neglect or waste of corporate assets, conflicts of interest or self-benefit, improper delegation of authority, harm done to third parties through tort (wrongful action) and/or breach of contract, and offenses against taxing authorities (Gelman, 1988). Even though board members may protect themselves through indemnification clauses and directors' and officers' liability insurance, they cannot escape charges of negligence or the wrath of communities and constituencies which feel that their trust has been betrayed.

RISK MANAGEMENT: GENERAL PRINCIPLES

Risk management is more than preventing bad things from happening. It implies an overarching consideration on the part of the organization with achieving its mission as efficiently and effectively as possible (Kurzman, 1995). Risk management is also not confined to business practices, per se, but extends to and incorporates how such practices impact on the main purpose of the residential treatment center: the provision of quality services and the assurance of positive outcomes for those served.

The overarching principle of risk management is the protection of those the organization serves, including its physical, human, and financial resources, through a process of evaluating and taking action to reduce risks to which they are exposed. Thus, risk management is an ongoing process, the impact of which is measurable through "smooth operations"–the lack of legal, regulatory, and professional problems.

The Council on Accreditation of Services to Families and Children (COA) is one accrediting body that has sought to articulate the role of the organization in risk management and to hold its accredited agencies to such standards. COA standards are particularly applicable to this discussion as the Council accredits residential treatment centers. Among the risk management mandates of COA (1997, Standard G6) are the following:

The organization has a process of evaluating and reducing its potential loss and liability which includes:

- Assigning the risk management function to a person whose job description includes responsibility for oversight of the risk management activities of the organization.
- Reporting to the governing body on the nature of risks involved, the steps to remedy them, and the need for bonding, self-insurance, or external coverage.
- Developing a process in which risks are identified and analyzed in terms of their nature, severity and frequency.
- Avoiding loss through prevention and risk reduction activities in combination with protection from risk.
- Evaluating and monitoring the effectiveness of the risk management function.

To implement the above-cited processes, the COA (1997, Standard G6.4.02, p. 42) standards specify that the organization's personnel are to be trained in:

- Personal safety measures.
- Techniques for deescalating conflict and handling emergencies.

- Guidelines for providing service to children and families with infectious diseases, including those who are HIV-positive or have AIDS, hepatitis, tuberculosis, or other similar problems.
- Other medical problems which may raise risks and may be present among the consumer group.

COA risk management standards (1997, Standard G6.4.05, G.4.06, G6.4.07, pp. 42-43) further specify the functions of the organization's management in this regard:

- The organization carries workers' compensation insurance and such other insurance as is deemed necessary based upon its evaluation of its risks and protects itself through means such as self-insurance, indemnification, participation in a risk-pooling trust, or external insurance coverage.
- The organization requires that all persons delegated the authority to sign checks, handle cash or contributions, or manage funds be bonded at the organization's expense or the organization maintains appropriate insurance coverage to cover losses which may be incurred.
- The organization discloses to its board members, trustees and/or officers, employees and volunteers the amount and type of coverage relevant to their need for protection which is provided on their behalf by the organization.

TYPES OF RISK MANAGEMENT

Financial Accountability

Organizations are expected to exercise "prudent fiscal management" (COA, 1997, p. 44). What, exactly, is "prudent"? According to the Council on Accreditation, indicators of prudent fiscal management include written operational procedures that comply with applicable legislation, regulation, or government directives and that address protection of assets of persons served, organizational accountability, and segregation of the funds, as applicable (COA, Standards G6, pp. 40-46). Other indicators include:

- Review and approval of the budget by the governing body prior to the beginning of the fiscal year.

- Review and approval of all material planned deviations from and revisions to the budget.
- Use of sound financial practices and generally accepted accounting principles in regard to income, expenditures, and financial accounting.
- Written operational procedures addressing internal accounting controls.
- Use of the accrual method of accounting.
- Assurances of timely tax payments to governmental taxing authorities, as required by law.
- Qualified staff to maintain the bookkeeping system.
- Maintenance of up-to-date accounting records.
- Systems to prevent or to detect fraud or abuses of the system, such as control, use, and review of the system by more than one person.
- Availability of an annual report of fiscal, statistical and service data which includes summary information regarding the organization's financial position.
- Performance of an audit of financial statements within the following year by an independent certified public accountant approved by the governing body.
- A review of the audit, financial statements, and any management letter by a financial or audit review committee, designated member of the governing body, or other agent of the governing body.
- Review and formal acceptance of the auditor's report by the board.
- Designation of a committee or agent of the board of agencies which invest their funds to oversee the investment and assure that practices conform to applicable legal and regulatory requirements.
- Ensure controls exist in regard to proper accounting of payroll costs (COA, Standard G6, pp. 40-46).

Assurance that these financial accountability standards are met is a particularly important function of the board in light of the recent media revelations of fiscal improprieties on the part of nonprofit agencies. Ethical and legal behavior on the part of both executives and board members is integral to the effective functioning of an organization (O'Neill, 1992). Good judgment can be suspended and replaced by high risk behavior in the search for funds. Even with an investment in greater oversight, such as more vigilant audits, it is incumbent upon nonprofit organizations to establish and maintain internal systems of accountability, a process that is the responsibility of the board of directors.

Service Accountability

Risk management is sometimes narrowly construed as behaving legally and overseeing the financial status of the organization. This conception is, however, too narrow. Service rendering agencies, such as residential treatment centers, need to ensure that the potential of risk is reduced for clients. Foremost, such considerations relate to the quality of the service environment and to accountability for the outcomes of the services rendered.

Table 1 highlights some of the COA residential service standards which exemplify areas over which the board must exercise oversight vigilance to manage organizational risk.

MANAGING RISK

As we approach the millennium, the political and social context in which residential treatment services are provided is changing significantly. Perhaps the most serious challenge from a risk management perspective is the overriding concern with the cost of care and efforts within government and the private sector to control costs. The mechanism for such control is managed care, which has been defined by the U.S. Department of Health and Human Services as: "an organized system of care which attempts to balance effectively access, quality, and cost by using utilization management, intensive case management, provider selection, and cost-containment methodologies" (Moss, 1995, p. 1).

The role of the board in risk management is of utmost importance within the context of an environment in which there is pressure to lower the levels of care (Edinburg & Cottler, 1995). Rigid precertification and recertification requirements; limitations on the length, duration and type of service; and restrictions on after-care services all potentially compromise the organization's service mission and its responsibilities to consumers and the public. The goal of cost effective-

TABLE 1. Sample Standards Related to the Risk Management Function in Residential Treatment Centers

Area of Risk	Standards
Organizational Environment	The organization carries out its programs in an environment which is safe, accessible, and appropriate for the needs of those served and with due regard for the rights and protections of those persons receiving services in an out-of-home environment.
	The organization is housed, equipped, and maintained in a manner which is suited to its program of services and which reflects the organization's positive regard for the persons it serves.
	The organization's premises and equipment are safe and functional for use by the persons served, personnel, and visitors.
	All physical facilities meet high standards for environmental quality and provide an effective context for delivery of services.
Legal Compliance	The organization makes its services accessible to its defined service population in full accord with all applicable federal and state legal and regulatory requirements.
	The organization is in compliance with applicable statutory requirements for its services.
Delivery of Services	The organization views services as part of a continuum of care and ensures that persons served receive care and treatment in a continuous manner with access to a coordinated, integrated system of settings, services, and care level based on individual need.
Behavioral Interventions	Positive behavioral methods and the use of environmental manipulation are used to promote constructive behaviors and to extinguish socially or personally detrimental or unacceptable behaviors.

TABLE 1 (continued)

Area of Risk	Standards
Behavioral Interventions (continued)	The organization's personnel are trained in appropriate forms of behavior management and use restrictive practices only under controlled conditions.
Medication	The residential center ensures that controls are in place governing the administration of medication.
Personnel	The service has qualified personnel who can meet the developmental and therapeutic needs of all persons accepted for care and services, their needs for protection and care, and the needs of their families for service.
Measuring Outcomes	The organization has an evaluation system in place to measure the outcomes of service delivery in regard to improving the psycho-social functioning of children and adults and achieving therapeutic treatment plan goals.
Quality Assurance	Group homes and residential centers examine the need for and appropriateness of service for persons served on a quarterly basis through conducting its own administrative review of: continued out-of-home care; efforts for family reunification; and the adequacy of efforts to preserve and continue treatment of the parent/family relationship when possible and in the best interest of the person served.

Source: Council on Accreditation of Services for Families and Children, Inc. (1997). *1997 standards for behavioral health care services and community support and educational services, United States edition.* New York: Author.

ness may mandate the shortest possible treatment stay, which may then compromise the responsibilities of the organization and make it vulnerable to legal liability. The board must balance these external requirements against the needs of the clients served.

A related and complicating factor concerns the continued diminishing of the federal government's fiscal role in human services. The trend to privatize human services, including residential services, continues, with the effect of emphasizing market considerations in service delivery. For-profit and nonprofit agencies are in a competitive position to offer services at the lowest costs. (See, for example, Gibelman & Demone, 1998.) More competitive cost structures may result in the elimination of some duplication and waste, but may also compromise the very areas of operations and services that are the concern of risk managers.

STRATEGIES

The reasons why a board of directors should embrace and engage in risk management are reasonably straightforward, as discussed above. Why, then, is managing risk not "a given" in nonprofit human service organizations? Three reasons stand out as factors. First, the leadership of an organization, both voluntary and paid staff, may lack information about risk and managing risk. Or, board and paid staff may assume that risk management is the responsibility of the other. Second, risk management involves some costs to the organization, typically in the form of time, effort, and insurance premiums. In this vein, the costs are ongoing and apparent, while potential losses are more amorphous and less tangible. Third, there has been an erroneous assumption of protected status. In fact, charitable organizations are no longer sacrosanct and good intentions no longer safeguard an organization from potential or actual liability. Nonprofit organizations are liable for the harm they cause to the same degree as for-profit enterprises. As one New Jersey court recently wrote:

> Due care is to be expected of all, and when an organization's negligent conduct injures another there should, in all justice and equity, be a basis for recovery without regard to whether the defendant is a private charity. (*Rupp v. Brookdale Baptist Church*, 1990, at 190)

Protected status is no longer afforded to the nonprofit (Kurzman, 1995; Tremper, 1994). Although some states have enacted various laws limiting the liability of charity organizations, immunity has disappeared in every state except Arkansas (Tremper, 1994). Limited liability may cap the amount of dollars for which an organization is liable or limit certain types of claims. Nevertheless, volunteers and staff are not immune from suit.

Clarifying Board-Staff Roles

The mandate of the board to provide risk management oversight involves a level of awareness of organizational operations, as well as the need for ongoing and vigilant oversight. This means that some of the problems that have surfaced in regard to the functioning of boards need to be addressed. Such problems include absentee governance, in which the elected board attends meetings but spends little time on board matters in between; board members who are unprepared for meetings and who fail to keep abreast of organizational developments; inability or unwillingness of a board to make decisions or a tendency to delay decisions; rubber stamping of the executives' recommendations without discussion; lack of clarification of the respective roles of board and staff; and/or board members' total isolation from staff, programs and clients (Gibelman, Gelman & Pollack, 1997).

Although the literature (e.g., Golensky, 1993; Howe, 1995; Kramer, 1985; Tropman, Johnson, & Tropman, 1992; Wiehe, 1978; Zander, 1993) is filled with contradictory statements about board-executive relations, it is clear that all must work together as partners. The executive director is delegated authority for the agency's day-to-day operations and for handling most personnel matters; however, laws and the agency's charter invest the board with the power and authority to make policy (Bubis & Dauber, 1987; Conrad & Glen, 1976; O'Connell, 1976). In other words, the ultimate responsibility for agency functioning and for the performance of the executive and staff resides with the board. The key, therefore, is the degree to which the board carries out its mandated role. Although the board can draw on the executive's expertise and knowledge, it cannot allow its legal responsibility to be diluted or co-opted by overdependence on paid staff (Gibelman, Gelman & Pollack, 1997).

Drucker (1990) maintains that nonprofits share in common the fact that many, if not most, suffer from malfunctions in their governance structure. Among the lessons Drucker offers is that board members need to take their job seriously and work hard at it. Too often, board members view their duties as merely perfunctory. Attendance at meetings may be inconsistent; lack of preparation for meetings may be even more common. Risk management may simply not be a concern.

Board Development

Unfortunately, many nonprofits do not provide formal training for board members to prepare them for their role. No assumptions should be made about the innate ability of even the most esteemed board members to understand and carry out their role. As Stephens (1995) commented:

> For some heretofore unexplained reason, many seasoned corporate executives, when they come to positions on nonprofit boards, feel compelled to leave their management, planning and fiscal training at the front door. The tendency is to "make allowances" where nonprofits are concerned, to give them "the benefit of the doubt." That attitude always breeds trouble. (p. 37)

Training should and must include the responsibilities of the board for risk management. The components of such training are identified in Table 2. Content should be specific to the circumstances and environment of each agency. However, certain legal obligations and ethical principles apply to all types of nonprofit human service organizations. In-service training for staff should also include these components to ensure that the voluntary leadership, management, and line staff are in accord regarding the importance of risk management vigilance and its impact on the day-to-day work and functioning of the agency. The focus of training should be on developing and applying those tools and materials pertinent to reducing legal vulnerability through prevention-oriented (risk management) practice.

Although formal board orientation is extremely important, it is insufficient. Board training must be ongoing and built in as a sched-

TABLE 2. Board, Management, and Staff Training in Risk Management: Suggested Content

Topic Area	Sample Content
Legal Obligations	Parameters of right to treatment Freedom of Information Act Federal Privacy Act Duty to warn (court decisions)
Confidentiality and Privileged Communication	Definitions–professional versus legal Informed consent Limitations to confidentiality Variations by state and content area (i.e., mandatory reporting of child abuse; involvement in divorce litigation)
Consequences for Violation	Contempt of Court Class actions Civil rights actions Indictment Professional sanctions (ethics)
Understanding Risks: Service Provision	Negligence Breach of duty (acts of omission or commission) Confidentiality and limitations Privileged communication Informed consent Conflict of interest Staff training and competence
Understanding Risks: Agency Oversight	Facilities Quality assurance Handling emergencies Disease prevention and control Insurance Financial checks and balances Staff qualifications
Resolution Process	Adjudication Mediation Suits Damages Settlements Professional standing

TABLE 2 (continued)

Topic Area	Sample Content

Managing Risk	Information needs
	    Federal, state and local laws
	    Standards of practice
	Consultation and supervision processes
	Record keeping
	Office procedure safeguards
	Quality assurance
	Adequacy of care
	Use of legal consultation
	Response to inquiries and/or complaints
	Liability insurance

Good Business Practices	Contracting (inter-organizational, government, consumers/families) Fee Setting Advertising Supervision, Consultation, and Case Review Termination of Services

uled, institutionalized event at least once a year. To the extent possible, joint board-staff training sessions should be normative, particularly in regard to mutual roles and responsibilities for risk management.

The failure to institute board development programs on a continuing basis often relates to the unwillingness of a board to invest scarce agency resources on itself. Instead, priority is afforded to using available dollars for organizational programs and services. This looks good to contributors and keeps administrative and governance costs down. However, such reasoning falls into the "penny wise, pound foolish" category. Systematic and ongoing board training is essential to knowledgeable governance.

Promoting and Rewarding Good Practice

The best form of risk management, particularly in regard to its service dimensions, is good practice. Reducing vulnerability to malpractice suits and professional liability risks suggests that principles of risk management must be incorporated into daily practice from a prevention perspective. From the client's first contact with the organization through termination of service, understanding of the law and regulations, of consumer rights, and of professional standards is essential (Houston-Vega, Nuehring, & Daguio, 1997). Staff must be held to the highest levels of accountability in regard to safeguarding privacy, confidentiality, and privileged communication. The organization must be vigilant about its billing practices. It must develop and implement documentation procedures and record-keeping systems that are responsive to the needs and demands of third party payers, accrediting bodies, government contract review mandates, and consumers. Although the chief executive officer has day-to-day responsibility for overseeing and supervising "good practice," it is, once again, the board that is ultimately accountable.

CONCLUSIONS

It cannot be assumed that nonprofit boards understand their role in risk management or are adequately prepared to assume it. Despite the proliferation of prescriptive literature on volunteer leadership recruitment, training, and retention, the fact remains that many boards are unwilling to invest in their own development, particularly in times of scarce resources. Good intentions and high ideals, however, are insufficient (Eisenberg, 1993).

If boards of directors do not take their responsibilities seriously, liability exposure will continue to increase. Watchdog agencies, such as the National Charities Information Bureau and the Better Business Bureau, are likely to become even more vigilant in their oversight roles, and with public sanction to do so. Similarly, the Internal Revenue Service is consistently observing the practices of nonprofit organizations and raising ongoing questions about whether protection of their distinct role continues to be warranted.

The best reason for managing risk is that it is in the interest of the organization and those it serves to do so. When risk is understood to extend to the quality and outcome of services as well as to the physical environment, per se, then the rationale for risk management may be seen as more compelling and more easily understood.

REFERENCES

Anthes, E.W. (1985). The board and the life of the organization: An overview. In E. Anthes, J. Crotin, & M. Jackson (Eds.), *The nonprofit board book: Strategies for organizational success* (rev. ed., 1-3). West Memphis and Hampton, AK: Independent Community Consultants.

Antler, S. (1985). *Child welfare at the crossroads: Professional liability.* Boston, MA: NASW, Massachusetts Chapter.

Axelrod, N.R. (1994). Board leadership and board development. In R.D. Herman & Associates. *The Jossey-Bass Handbook of Nonprofit Leadership & Management,* 119-136. San Francisco, CA: Jossey-Bass.

Besharov, D. (1985). *The vulnerable social worker.* Silver Spring, MD: National Association of Social Workers.

Bryant, Y., & Korsak, A. (1988). Who is the risk manager and what does he do? *Hospitals, 52,* 42-43.

Bubis, G.B., & Dauber, J. (1987). The delicate balance–Board-staff relations. *Journal of Jewish Communal Service, 63*(3), 187-196.

Conrad, W., & Glen, W. (1976). *The effective voluntary board of directors.* Boulder, CO: National Center for Voluntary Action.

Council on Accreditation of Services for Families and Children, Inc. (1997). *1997 standards for behavioral health care services and community support and educational services, United States edition.* New York: Author.

Drucker, P.F. (1990). Lessons for successful nonprofit governance. *Nonprofit Management & Leadership, 1,* (1), 7-14.

Edinburg, G.M., & Cottler, J.M. (1995). Managed care. In R.L. Edwards (ed.-in-chief), *Encyclopedia of social work* (19th ed., 1635-1641). Washington, DC: NASW Press.

Eisenberg, P. (1993, July 13). Press coverage sends a message to non-profits: Clean up your act. *Chronicle of Philanthropy,* 41-42.

Gelman, S.R. (1983). The board of directors and agency accountability. *Social Casework, 64*(2), 83-91.

Gelman, S.R. (1988). Roles, responsibilities, and liabilities of agency boards. In M. Janicki, M.W. Krause, & M. Seltzer (Eds.), *Community residences for persons with developmental disabilities: Here to stay* (57-68). Baltimore: Paul H. Brookes.

Gelman, S.R. (1992). Risk management through client access to case records. *Social Work, 37*(1), 73-79.

Gelman, S.R. (1995). Boards of directors. In R. Edwards (Ed.-in-Chief), *Encyclopedia of Social Work* (19th ed., 305-312). Washington, DC: NASW Press.

Gelman, S.R., Gibelman, M., Pollack, D., & Schnall, D. (1996). Philanthropic boards of directors on the line: Roles, realities and prospects. *Journal of Jewish Communal Service, 72*(3), 185-194.

Gibelman, M., Gelman, S.R., & Pollack, D. (1996). The credibility of nonprofit boards: A view from the 1990s. *Administration in Social Work, 21* (2) 29-40.

Gibelman, M. & Demone, H.W., Jr. (Eds.) (1998). *The privatization of human services: Policy and practice issues.* New York: Springer.

Golensky, M. (1993). The board-executive relationship in nonprofit organizations: Partnership or power struggle? *Nonprofit Management and Leadership, 4*(2), 177-191.

Hanson, P.L., & Marmaduke, C.T. (1972). The board member-decision maker for the nonprofit corporation. Sacramento, CA: HAN/MAR Publications.

Houston-Vega, M.K., Nuehring, E.M., & Daguio, E.R. (1997). *Prudent practice: A guide for managing malpractice risk.* Washington, DC: NASW Press.

Howe, F. (1995). *Welcome to the board.* San Francisco, CA: Jossey-Bass.

Joseph, M.V. (1989, October 14). Presentation at the 1989 NASW Annual Conference, "At Risk: Legal Vulnerability and What to Do About It." San Francisco, CA.

Kearns, K.P. (1996). *Managing for accountability.* San Francisco, CA: Jossey-Bass.

Kramer, R.M. (1985). Toward a contingency model of board-executive relations. *Administration in Social Work, 9*(3), 15-33.

Kurzman, P.A. (1995). Professional liability and malpractice. In R.L. Edwards (Ed.-in-chief), *Encyclopedia of Social Work* (19th ed., 1921-1927). Washington, DC: NASW Press.

Leifer, J.C., & Glomb, M.B. (1992). *The legal obligations of nonprofit boards: A guidebook for board members.* Washington, DC: National Center for Nonprofit Boards.

Mitton, D.G. (1974). Utilizing the board of trustees: A unique structural design. *Child Welfare, 53*(6), 345-351.

Monagle, J.F. (1985). *Risk management: A guide for health care professionals.* Rockville, MD: Aspen.

Moss, S. (1995). *Purchasing managed care services for alcohol and other drug treatment.* Technical assistance publication series, No. 16, Vol. III. Rockville, MD: U.S. Department of Health and Human Services Publication No. (SMA) 95-3040.

O'Connell, B. (1976). *Effective leadership in voluntary organizations.* New York: Association Press.

O'Neill, M. (1992). Ethical dimensions of nonprofit administration. *Nonprofit Management & Leadership, 3*(2), 199-213.

Roswell, V.A. (1988). Professional liability: Issues for behavior therapists in the 1980s and 1990s. *The Behavior Therapist, 11*(8), 163-171.

Rupp v. Brookdale Baptist Church, 577 A.2d 188 (N.J.Super.A.D. 1990).

Siciliano, J., & Spiro, G. (1992). The unclear status of nonprofit directors: An empirical survey of director liability. *Administration in Social Work, 16*(1), 69-80.

Tremper, C. (1989). *Reconsidering legal liability and insurance for nonprofit organizations.* Lincoln, NB: Law College Education Services, Inc.

Tremper, C. (1994). Risk management. In R.D. Herman & Associates (Eds.), *The Jossey-Bass Handbook of Nonprofit Leadership and Management,* 485-508. San Francisco, CA: Jossey-Bass.

Tropman, E., Johnson, H.R., & Tropman, E. (1992). *Committee management in human services* (2nd edition). Chicago, IL: Nelson Hall.

Wiehe, V.R. (1978). Role expectations among agency personnel. *Social Work, 22,* 270-274.

Zander, A. (1993). *Making boards effective.* San Francisco, CA: Jossey-Bass.

The Changing Role of Trustees
in Fund Raising
for Residential Treatment Centers

David Kirk, DMin
Judy T. Lindsey, MS, CFRE

SUMMARY. There is an abundance of literature about the role of trustees in preserving and advancing the missions of their organizations. Numerous resources exist on governance, stewardship, volunteer leadership development, and trustees' roles in fund raising. These contributions to the field have affected the ethics and practices of many not-for-profit organizations.

Current environmental changes mandate additional discussion on ways that board and staff can work together to assure the viability of their organizations. Generous government funding played a pivotal role in the growth of many residential treatment centers for several decades. Therefore, the search for philanthropic support often became secondary. However, dramatic decreases in government funding, closer regulatory scrutiny, and charities' increased accountability to donors has changed that landscape. This dictates a review of the manner in which organizations educate their trustees about their roles in fund raising.

Based on the authors' experience with their organization's two-year journey with this process, the article explores: (1) the effective involvement of trustees in strategic planning and program policy as they are related to fund raising, and (2) the partnership between trustees and staff in creating an organizational spirit of mission-driven support. *[Article copies available for a fee from The Haworth Document Delivery Service: 1-800-342-9678. E-mail address: getinfo@haworthpressinc.com <Website: http://www.haworthpressinc.com>*

[Haworth co-indexing entry note]: "The Changing Role of Trustees in Fund Raising for Residential Treatment Centers." Kirk, David, and Judy T. Lindsey. Co-published simultaneously in *Residential Treatment for Children & Youth* (The Haworth Press, Inc.) Vol. 16, No. 4, 1999, pp. 39-50; and: *The New Board: Changing Issues, Roles and Relationships* (ed: Nadia Ehrlich Finkelstein, and Raymond Schimmer) The Haworth Press, Inc., 1999, pp. 39-50. Single or multiple copies of this article are available for a fee from The Haworth Document Delivery Service [1-800-342-9678, 9:00 a.m. - 5:00 p.m. (EST). E-mail address: getinfo@haworthpressinc.com].

KEYWORDS. Nonprofits, boards, fund raising, strategic planning, capital campaign

Literature on the nonprofit sector is rich with information about the role of trustees in preserving and advancing the missions of the organizations they support. Indeed, numerous resources exist on governance, stewardship, volunteer leadership development, trustees' roles and responsibilities, fund raising and much more. These contributions have shaped ethics and practices, and have improved the ways that organizations in the third sector conduct business.

However, the dramatic environmental changes that are affecting nonprofits today stimulate additional discussion regarding the mutual responsibility of board and staff in securing the future of their organizations. For several decades, government funding of nonprofit organizations has played a critical role in their growth. In many instances, the availability of public support has precluded the need to develop and diversify sources of private financial resources, including voluntary contributions from individuals, corporations and foundations. However, that landscape has been altered significantly with decreased government funding, closer regulatory scrutiny, controversial incidents that have affected the public's trust in charitable organizations, and donors' requests for accountability. All of these factors compel us to review the ways we involve and educate trustees about their significance in the life and work of our organizations. When it comes to fund raising—the most visible role a trustee can assume—the education process must extend beyond training on traditional gift solicitation techniques and include their deep involvement in the actualization of the organization's mission.

In his contemporary and acclaimed text, *Achieving Excellence in Fund Raising* (1991), Henry Rosso states that an organization may claim a *right* to raise money by asking for the tax deductible gift. Instead, it must earn the *privilege* of raising money by demonstrating its responsiveness to needs, the worthiness of its programs, and the good stewardship exercised by its governing body.

Rosso's operative word is "privilege." One might consider this privilege as the organization's obligation not to violate the public's trust in the way it communicates its needs, manages its programs, and most important, keeps its trustees and other constituents informed of its challenges as well as its accomplishments. The latter becomes mandatory in preparing any trustee to become a credible messenger of the organization's good work, an advocate for its cause, a recruiter of new board leadership and a solicitor of gifts.

New developments challenge us as we address these issues today. The most apparent is the decrease in government support. A study which was conducted among 108 diverse nonprofit organizations revealed that nonprofit organizations would have to increase their private revenues by 70% over seven years to maintain stable service levels. From 2001 to 2002, these organizations would have to increase voluntary contributions by 124% (Melendez 1995, *unpublished presentation*). This dramatic reality is intensified especially as child welfare agencies attempt to cope with more complex needs exhibited by the children, such as increased need for psychotropic medications; services needed for drug exposed infants and the long-term impact on their behavior; fiscal impact of performance-based contracts and valid outcome measures of service; the managed care environment; a retooling of staff to meet the therapeutic needs of children entering residential treatment who are older and more aggressive; and, the quest for more cost-effective services using briefer, yet clinically responsive, treatment modalities.

This complexity challenges our ability to communicate all dimensions of need to trustees. It is no longer sufficient to present mere client statistics and vague yet empathetic descriptions of programs. Staff must strive to effectively weave trustees into the organization's cycle of planning and problem solving as they weather the storm of contemporary funding challenges. Being equipped with the facts, participating in planning, and making important governance decisions should be incorporated in a way that creates organizational synergy and results in commitment, an increased understanding of issues, and informed action by trustees.

In this regard, the service delivery becomes the heart of the organization while the governance and policy action of trustees become the conscience. It is the latter that will serve to protect the integrity and future existence of programs as organizations face hazy horizons. How this translates into an increase in resources–volunteer, financial, and in-kind–is the challenge of the journey.

THE HIDDEN CASE FOR SUPPORT

There are reasons why organizations and services come into existence. These reasons become the core of the nonprofit's case for support. Experienced fund raisers know how powerful a good case for support can be. The case is the document of definition demonstrating that significant needs are being addressed by the institution. It also should illustrate the organization's unique capacity to fulfill those needs. That fulfillment is stated in terms of the organization's impact on its primary customer, the child. Service value to its secondary constituents, such as immediate or extended family members, foster parents or adoptive parents who receive indirect benefits from the organization's programs, also can be highlighted. Trustees, too, are included as secondary constituents because through their participation they receive intangible benefits such as satisfaction, a sense of civic pride, and recognition, to name a few. Last, but certainly not least, the value of the institution's work to its tertiary sector, that is the community-at-large, must be revealed. The tertiary sector includes sources which may have the capacity to provide major gifts, such as foundations and corporations and individuals who do not have a direct relationship with the organization but have a vested interest in how it is contributing to their local community or society in general.

These distinctions are important when discussing residential services because in most cases, neither the organization's primary "customers"–the children who receive the most immediate and direct benefits of service–nor secondary "customers" (their parents who receive the indirect benefit of having their child provided with care) have the capacity to provide financial support. Therefore, the case has to be powerful enough to extend beyond them to tertiary constituents such as potential donors and demonstrate why they should embrace the mission of the organization and support its work. This is a tall task because the case should initially move the potential donor to a point of readiness to give, and secondarily, be compelling enough to stimulate generous and continuous giving. The case, therefore, is not just a list of facts, but a clear statement of the impact of the organization's service, its vital use to its community and how it is addressing issues that extend beyond its institutional walls (Alford 1991, *unpublished presentation*).

If the residential treatment center is part of a multi-service agency, the case for the residential service becomes a "hidden" case within the institution's comprehensive case for support. For example, a child welfare agency's overall case for support may clearly illustrate how its programs, from prevention to intervention, are protecting children, supporting families and thereby providing all with services that will lead to a productive future. The case within that case (i.e., residential treatment services) could provide a finely tuned account of how that specific service is an essential building block of the agency's overall mission. Since confidentiality requirements restrict the disclosure of residents' identity, the case must create a vivid picture of life within the walls of the residential treatment center and bring the reader information that provides rationality in support of the emotional need for giving. Yet, there are other windows of understanding that can be opened by the "hidden" case for support.

There is opportunity to embed information in the case that reinforces the business logic of the operations, past accomplishments, history of service patterns, marketplace competition, and measures of accountability. All of these components treat the reader as an insider and provide contemporary perspectives that are unique to residential treatment centers today. Given the fact that residential services are less visible to the public, such information can provide assurances about management's and program staff's capacity to deliver quality service, even in the midst of change. While enhancing the reader's sensibilities, this creates a framework for sound decision making. An example might be the organization's fiscal and program plan to adjust to changes in public funding and, within that context, make service changes to serve a changing client population.

Concurrently, the case becomes the tool that helps trustees to better understand the center's needs and empowers them to participate in substantive planning for the organization's future. In that regard, they become not only insiders but also true advisors and stakeholders. Most importantly, the case statement should instill within the trustee a heightened sense of pride in affiliation with the organization. In this climate of change, we must equip trustees with sound measures of accountability. These measures are the bases on which they can and will promote the organization within their circle of contacts.

This is a paradigm shift from the traditional orientation and training, and continuing education of trustees. Typically, the routine introduction has been a tour of the facility. It has been a hands-on experience that clearly shows the need, both capital and programmatic. Next, there may have been carefully structured interactions between selected residents of the facility and staff. Another approach has been time limited or long-term involvement along the dimensions of specific volunteer activities or special projects, such as holiday activities or special recreational excursions. These activities do get to the heart of the service with a hands-on approach.

However, elevating these activities to another level of participation is an important transition. A construct for consideration is to align the trustees' education process with a developmental model of fund raising maturation for the organization. Utilizing a paradigm presented by The Alford Group (1988), trustees' experience might be aligned with fund raising maturation as shown in Table 1.

Questions, then, that staff and trustees should be prepared to address might include the following: How does one measure the positive impact of therapeutic intervention in the life of a child? How does one guarantee the outcomes of such treatment? What does the organization expect to accomplish at the end of its work in the life of a child in residential treatment? How is the request for voluntary dollars justified when the residential treatment center historically has been heavily funded by government contracts? How will the organization demonstrate its return on the donor's investment? What financial management adjustments will the residential treatment center make if the needs of children change? Are there strategic alliances that could be formed with other providers, both for-profit and nonprofit, that would lead to more efficient operations? How does the organization translate the desired results into terms that a trustee who is soliciting funds for the organization can comprehend and explain to others?

ANOTHER FORM OF PLANNING

A common staff technique in working with trustees has been to provide training on gift solicitation. The training material has included a list of reasons why one should support the organization, often presented in isolation of the trustees' involvement in planning for an organization's future. While this approach may be efficient and digestible, it negates the power of inclusion, thereby reducing benefits that can be derived from broadening trustees' understanding of why funds need to

TABLE 1

STAGE OF FUND RAISING MATURATION	COMMON BELIEFS	TRUSTEE EXPERIENCE
I. PRODUCT STAGE	"The residential center is a good reputable institution. People should contribute based on its history of helping children. If asked, donors will give. The institution is worthy."	Facility tour; selected involvement with residents illustrating quality of program; client success stories.
II. SALES STAGE	"There must be many people who are sympathetic to causes related to children. We just have to find them and ask for support."	Selected constituents, e.g., donor prospects, are invited for special tours or presentations about the facility.
III. MARKETING STAGE	"There is increased competition for funding and new service delivery challenges. The organization must analyze its position in the market place of residential service providers and concentrate on marketing its core competencies (e.g., success with specific resident populations and cost effectiveness of service) which result in measurable outcomes that can be presented to those whose interests best match ours. The organization must promote its unique selling propositions."	Trustee involvement on program policy committee to examine program direction, impact from public policy changes, outcome measures to evaluate market value of service to referral sources; review of fiscal reports to determine cost/benefit ratio; examination of inherent value of service vs. costs; exploration of strategic alliances with other providers in the same market; long-term capital and operational planning; adjusting services to respond to managed care.

Note. Adapted by authors.

be solicited for this organization. Understanding a specific organization is of particular importance for trustees who sit on several boards.

An effective, educational tool for creating this understanding is a carefully crafted long range planning process that involves both board and key staff in the activities. Through a carefully planned process, trustees' importance in the life and work of the organization can be emphasized, staff can become exposed to perspectives that are not part of their daily thinking, and all can reach consensus on the strategic goals of the organization and the resources that will be needed to achieve those goals. Without such a process, the fund raising role of trustees becomes artificially separated from the programmatic heart of the organization, and trustees (as solicitors) can be left ill-equipped to represent the full case of the organization to a prospective donor. The planning process can effectively create a level of understanding that creates a comfort level for trustees to speak to others about the organization.

For example, it may not be realistic to expect trustees to be fully knowledgeable about program details of the residential facility. However, through participation in a productive long range planning process, they will become armed with a high level of confidence, and the prospective donor may be assured of the program's integrity, feasibility and accountability. These authors have seen the latter approach used by trustees in creating interest in a prospective donor and as an effective way to recruit new board members. This approach also assures the trustee that his or her time and talent are just as important as a monetary gift, thereby lessening the feeling that the trustee's only value to the organization is to give and/or raise money.

The final product should not be just a written document or new mission statement, but the process outcomes must include a sense of ownership, vision, reaffirmation of organizational strengths and commitment to quality. These process outcomes should create an invigorating sense of purpose and infuse both board and staff with clarity of direction–a direction that should serve as an anchor that is revisited regularly and that will help the organization withstand anticipated or unanticipated challenges of the changing external environment. It should also solidify the partnership and open communication with staff if future decisions become difficult.

In terms of content, at a minimum, the strategic planning process should cover the key areas of examination–program policy, human resources, financial development, and board development. However, in the case of residential treatment centers, the program component might include areas that need additional examination such as responding to the managed care environment, adapting operations for a different population with more severe needs, capital changes to meet new client needs or regulatory standards, development of staff skills in new treatment modalities, and the acquisition of resources to make this happen. Of course, the latter would require that the plan carefully address the financial needs of the treatment center within the context of the total organization.

While a number of models for this process may be adopted, it is important that it not become one that is so driven by staff that it discourages or devalues input from the trustees. Staff must be willing to address difficult questions that are asked by the trustees, and trustees should bring their external perspectives to the process that staff may overlook. It is the reciprocity of the process that enriches the organization and results in the plan that sets the course for the future. It should be noted that everyone involved needs to approach the process in a manner that creates a mission driven direction for the organization. Staff should exit from the process with a plan that guides the operations and trustees should depart with a tool that allows them to exercise their governance responsibilities in the areas of program policy, board recruitment and financial management.

The process stimulates trustees' strategic thinking beyond annual operating support to major capital initiatives and, most importantly, to endowment building. This thinking can be extended into setting multi-year fund raising goals that not only reflect the need for annual operating support but also focus on ways to diversify and/or expand the mix of available funds. For example, does the organization want to systematically decrease its percentage of government funding while increasing its percentage of voluntary contributions and investment income? Are there opportunities to create mission-related earned income ventures without jeopardizing the charitable tax-exempt status of the organization? Should the organization plan for a capital campaign that is strategically enriched with a fund raising component to build an endowment?

The latter financial considerations, absent the underpinning of a sound program direction, could result in empty gestures to engage trustees while asking for a considerable commitment of time and resources. Genuinely engaging trustees in long-range planning will make their expertise available for the process of identifying salient needs and applying necessary resources. In many ways, the *process* of planning becomes almost more important than the plan itself. Nothing can replace, in quality and substance, the value of genuine involvement.

AN EXPERIENCE IN PROGRESS

In 1993, the trustees of Children's Home & Aid Society of Illinois completed an overwhelmingly successful, multi-million dollar campaign that resulted in the construction of a state-of-the-art residential treatment center for severely emotionally disturbed children. The positive campaign results, which exceeded the goal by 25%, created a climate of volunteer involvement. However, within a year of the campaign's end, it became apparent that the external environment was shifting. Children with more complex needs were being referred to the facility. This potentially affected treatment modalities, staffing, and costs. By 1995, the trustees recognized that to preserve the benefits of the capital campaign new plans needed to be developed in order to adapt to the external environment. The collective and individual thoughts and actions of the immediate past chairman, chief executive officer, and new board chairman, whose platform was partially based on the urgency of the need, was the impetus for a strategic planning process with strong trustee involvement. The executive team realized that the strategic, capital and campaign gains were approaching obsolescence in relationship to some of the following factors:

- Escalating violence in society resulting in increased economic and educational disparity leading to increased poverty with commensurate increases in child abuse and neglect.
- Increased substance abuse as a major contributor to abuse and neglect of children and breakdown of the family structure.
- Paradigm shifts moving service delivery from intervention and remediation to prevention.
- Pressure to create a managed care behavioral health care delivery system in an effort to contain cost while ensuring quality care.
- Reductions in government support but the continued increase in state-mandated services for children.
- Changing referral priorities, i.e., children presenting more complex problems thus requiring the organization to re-visit its core competencies and implement plans for staff development to assure effective and appropriate care.
- Accelerating technological advances creating an information-based society and greater access to information about nonprofit organizations by the public.

- New welfare reform initiatives, of which the impact on children remains unknown.

Rather than approach these changes with a sense of insecurity, Children's Home & Aid Society's long-range planning process was utilized as an opportunity to involve trustees in examining the organization's core competencies in an effort to prepare for the future.

By the end of the next fiscal year, serious discussions were underway regarding our organization's largest residential facility. Statewide, the number of children in group living arrangements plummeted and as a reflection of this trend, the residential treatment center experienced fewer referrals. More and more children between ten and sixteen years of age were being referred. Historically, this residential treatment center had served children between five and fourteen years of age. Also, just one year earlier only 30% of the children referred to the facility were on psychotropic medications. That percentage rose dramatically to 70% in less than twelve months.

The long range planning process had prepared trustees and management for these changes, but it was not expected that they would occur at such an accelerated pace. Equipped with information derived from the long range planning process, the board's program policy and finance committee members became astute advisors. While remaining mindful of the financial impact of this trend, their sensitivity to and understanding of these challenges provided a balanced platform for discussion and planning.

By mid-year, the trustees sanctioned the following short-term program and budget modifications recommended by the Center's administrator while other long-term strategies continued to be explored: (1) implement an expanded program model, increasing medical and psychiatric services and retain a part-time medical director, and (2) proceed with a short-term consolidation of residential operations into four living units rather than five.

One trustee introduced the Center to a private adoption agency in need of temporary space. As a result, an unused unit of the residential center secured a temporary tenant whose rent offset some of the loss of revenue. Concurrently, staff continued to build internal capacity to accommodate older and more seriously disturbed youth.

One challenge is that this shift in population may or may not be accepted by the community where the treatment center is located. Given this as a possibility, an option might be to form a strategic alliance with a service provider that has a successful track record with the type of youth referred. This provider's service experience could be positioned in a way to ease community concerns regarding any changes in the treatment center's population.

Mixed use of the building is another consideration yet to be explored. For example, a business arrangement with a for-profit or non-profit continuing care residential center for senior citizens could be entertained. Children's Home & Aid Society of Illinois might propose that one floor be utilized for one of its programs, such as day care. Such a collaboration would allow for some creative intergenerational programs that might be of interest to private philanthropic sources of support.

Regardless of the outcome, trustees and staff will need to work in partnership to develop strategies to educate donors, especially those who gave substantial gifts to build the facility. As "investors" and "stakeholders," they will need to learn about changes in the building's use and its programs. Communicating the ways in which their campaign gifts have empowered Children's Home & Aid Society of Illinois to adapt to contemporary environmental changes while preserving its legacy of quality service will require careful thought.

Cultivating the donors' understanding of how their contributions have helped the organization weather the storms of change may be difficult. However, having trustees, many of whom were campaign contributors themselves, participate in this process should facilitate the achievement of that goal. Building a new case for support with trustees who have been intimately involved in the process of change can have a significant impact on the life of an organization.

REFERENCES

Alford, J.R. (1991) Are You Ready for Campaign? Chicago: unpublished presentation, United Way of Lake County.

Benuska, M. & Lindsey, J.T. (September, 1997) Wanted Development Officers, Chicago: unpublished presentation, Midwest Regional Conference, National Society of Fund Raising Executives-Chicago Chapter.

Lord, J.G. (1987). The Raising of Money–Thirty-Five Essentials Every Trustee Should Know, Cleveland: Third Sector Press.

Melendez, S.E. (August, 1995) Ethics, Stewardship, and Mission. Indianapolis: unpublished presentation, 8th Annual Symposium, Indiana University Center on Philanthropy.

Rosso, H.A. & Associates (1991). Achieving Excellence in Fund Raising, San Francisco: Jossey-Bass Publishers.

Boards of Directors and Agencies Adapting to Managed Care

Mildred B. Shapiro, MA

SUMMARY. Boards of Directors of not-for-profit children's agencies need to become familiar with the risk involved in the new environment of managed care. Efficiency and cost-sensitivity have not been the hallmark of such agencies in the past. Under managed care, Boards need to be more concerned with the bottom line. Managed care offers much promise for better coordinated community-based care. However, critics are concerned that the poor and chronically mentally ill have not fared well in a managed care setting. Changing incentives may lead to reduction or withholding of services. Continuing education is a must for Board members if the agency is to survive and thrive, and take advantage of the opportunities offered by managed care. *[Article copies available for a fee from The Haworth Document Delivery Service: 1-800-342-9678. E-mail address: getinfo@haworthpressinc.com <Website: http://www.haworthpressinc.com>]*

KEYWORDS. Nonprofits, boards, managed care, residential treatment

The managed care revolution is gathering momentum even as some critics claim it is running out of steam. The environment is changing radically for children's services, health and welfare agencies. Indeed, even as many such nonprofit agencies are struggling to adjust and cope with the restraints of managed care, one executive of a major health maintenance organization (HMO), prone to hyperbole, described managed care as "a product whose time has come and gone"

[Haworth co-indexing entry note]: "Boards of Directors and Agencies Adapting to Managed Care." Shapiro, Mildred B. Co-published simultaneously in *Residential Treatment for Children & Youth* (The Haworth Press, Inc.) Vol. 16, No. 4, 1999, pp. 51-62; and: *The New Board: Changing Issues, Roles and Relationships* (ed: Nadia Ehrlich Finkelstein, and Raymond Schimmer) The Haworth Press, Inc., 1999, pp. 51-62. Single or multiple copies of this article are available for a fee from The Haworth Document Delivery Service [1-800-342-9678, 9:00 a.m. - 5:00 p.m. (EST). E-mail address: getinfo@haworthpressinc.com].

(Freudenheim 1997). But clearly managed care, in an evolving form, is here to stay. Such are the dynamics of the industry that market forces and contracts are replacing government regulation, and providers of child care services will be learning the real meaning of the word *risk*. Children and family agencies, having accepted contractual responsibility to provide comprehensive care, may necessarily become purchasers of services that are not within their legal authorization or professional competence, all for a fixed periodic fee paid to the agency. This assumption of risk could be a rude introduction to the world of capitation.

BOARDS OF DIRECTORS

Responsibilities

In this very dynamic environment, how do boards of directors of nonprofit children's services agencies do their job when most come to these positions very well-intentioned but ill-prepared for the tasks ahead? Even in a stable environment, being an effective board member does not come naturally, but requires ongoing education and instruction. For board members with prior experience, there is no automatic transference from having served on a school board to serving on a children's services agency board.

Being a board member of a nonprofit children's services agency or any other similar board means setting policy or direction–generally. But specifically, governing boards are responsible for attending meetings; monitoring the effectiveness of existing policies; hiring and delegating management authority to an administrator; planning for the year ahead, ensuring the financial stability and survival of the organization (including annual budget approval, contracting for an independent audit and controlling investment policies); engaging in long-range planning with ongoing adjustments, and being an advocate for the agency in the community.

Unlike a for-profit organization whose focus is the bottom line, and whose accountability is to stockholders, not-for-profit organizations are judged by the services they provide, and are accountable to their various constituencies, e.g., troubled children, their families, government and legislative officials. That is not to say that financial stability is not a significant responsibility of nonprofit board members who

must participate in attracting contributions for the financing of programs, in addition to overseeing revenue from services performed and
management of costs.

Board members, in their oversight role, need to assure that the
agency is not standing still, but is on the cutting edge, moving with the
dynamics of the social, political and economic environment. With so
many philosophical, legislative, and marketplace changes occurring in
child welfare, mental health and health care, meeting this challenge
could be a high-wire act.

Life Before Managed Care

In a fee-for-service, open-ended funding environment, most children's services agencies have dealt with a variety of government agencies at the federal, state and local levels (including Medicaid), school
districts, and those offices with jurisdiction for social services, mental
health, and health. In some regions of the country, children's services,
health and welfare agencies may be supported totally by membership
organizations or by charitable foundations.

In addition to caring for Medicaid clients, nonprofit agencies have
served the working poor or the large numbers of uninsured who are
deemed ineligible for Medicaid, those who cannot afford to purchase
health insurance on their own, and whose employers do not cover
them or their families. Agencies have been able to serve this population through cross-subsidies from a variety of funding streams (except
from those government programs where funds are restricted). Revenues and costs were often predictable from year-to-year, with the usual
adjustments for inflation and new programs.

But nonprofit agencies in the past, and possibly the present as well,
have not had a reputation for efficiency and hard-nosed business practices. They have not aggressively ferreted out inefficiencies, or reduced unnecessary services. They have passively suffered missed appointments and loss of productivity as a necessary cost of doing
business. And incentives under fee for service encouraged use of the
most expensive modality for the longest period of time. Cost sensitivity was not a burning issue.

The Pathways to Managed Care

Managed care which, for the most part, is capitation-based and
provides for an annual set fee per person per year for a defined pack-

age of benefits, reverses the incentives of fee for service. Since the agency will receive a global fee, irrespective of the amount or type of services rendered, it becomes prudent to focus on doing less instead of more. Cost-effectiveness for the desired outcome needs to become the norm.

The growth of managed care in the private sector has been phenomenal. Over 70 percent of insured Americans are now enrolled in some form of managed care as major corporations have made health care cost containment a high priority. Government health programs, also wrestling with skyrocketing health expenditures, have adopted managed care as a strategy to rein in costs. Consequently, Medicaid managed care has experienced exceptional growth as more and more states receive federal waivers to mandate the enrollment of Medicaid recipients into managed care organizations. Medicaid managed care grew from 9.5 percent to 40.1 percent of total Medicaid enrollment in the 1991-1996 period. However, about one-third of Medicaid managed care enrollees remain in Primary Care Case Management where services are paid for on the traditional fee-for-service arrangement. Children account for more than half of the Medicaid population, making them a focal point of managed care.

Agencies which typically dealt with a very small percentage of traditional (Blue Cross/Blue Shield and commercial indemnity) health insurance companies and a greater percentage of Medicaid clients are now finding themselves engaged in contract negotiations with a wider and wider pool of managed care organizations (MCOs) demanding discounted rates.

But typically, MCOs have enrolled employed healthy populations, with little experience in dealing with the chronically mentally ill. The ability of HMOs to provide for seriously emotionally disturbed (SED) children and adolescents without the appropriate expert staff to treat these young new enrollees remains questionable.

Because of these concerns, the Health Care Financing Administration, in its 1115 demonstration waiver proposals, exempted children with special needs from the broad mandate of enrolling all Medicaid recipients into MCOs (along with other special needs populations) and provided for separate plans designated as *mental health special needs plans (MHSNPs)* for SED children. A second type of waiver available to the states, called a Section 1915(b) "Freedom of Choice" waiver, allows states to mandate managed care for Medicaid enrollees, but beneficiaries are required to have a choice of health plans. Such waivers have been granted to 42 states as of January 1997, while 1115 waivers were granted to 16 states. The outcome of these programs is still indeterminate.

The scarcity of high quality mental health care is not unique to MCOs. A recent study by the Center for Studying Health System Change (1997) reported that the overwhelming majority of primary care physicians, i.e., family practitioners, internists and pediatricians have difficulty in obtaining high quality mental health care (both inpatient and outpatient) for their patients. Among their conclusions: *The widespread initiation of managed care behavioral health programs also could affect the availability of mental health care.*

This paucity of high quality mental health resources coupled with the high cost of these services in acute care hospitals puts nonprofit children's services agencies in a unique competitive position, offering quality specialized services at relatively attractive prices.

This transition to managed care will require a change in thinking or philosophy on the part of the board and agency staff, with more emphasis on the bottom line. Programs will need to be self-sustaining. Boards will have to review each program from a profit/loss perspective. Cash flow needs of the agency will become more critical as lending institutions are loathe to extend credit in a risky environment. Subsidies to hard-driving for-profit insurance plans may no longer be possible.

Nonprofit agencies which are thinly capitalized will need to better predict their costs in a higher risk environment where program changes ultimately affect costs. For example, shortened lengths of stay under capitation payments will increase cost per day.

Nonprofit agencies do not have the reserves to cushion a program's unanticipated losses. Subsidies will no longer be available in an environment dominated by managed care.

It is doubtful that many nonprofit agencies, particularly those on a shaky fiscal foundation, would rush to fully capitate all their services. It is more likely that children's services agencies will move slowly, under a partial capitation arrangement for child welfare services, while others may assume the risk for behavioral health. The more daring and more financially secure may undertake a full capitation program (possibly with some carve-outs), for behavioral health, child welfare, and education.

The Promise of Managed Care

One of the major concerns of boards of directors in children's services agencies is the quality of care delivered to those children receiving services. Managed care, which creates a sensitivity to costs while focusing on outcomes, can offer the following:

- Higher value on prevention programs as a way to decrease future costs.
- Reduced bias for institutional care.
- Easy access to a mental health professional who knows the child, and provides more appropriate services in a less restrictive environment in the community.
- Continuity and integration of a broad spectrum of community-based-services.
- Coordinated service systems, such as mental health, physical health, child protective and child welfare, and education.
- Integrated home-based services with children, their families, and collaborative relationships with the providers who serve them.

Some advocacy organizations, among them the Child Welfare League of America (CWLA) and the Institute for Family-Centered Care, have developed guidelines to assist MCOs and family advocates in the design of new systems of health and welfare integration. CWLA operates a Managed Care Institute for Children's Services, promoting best practices for cost-effective quality care for all children's services in a managed care environment. The promise is there as well as the opportunity for technical assistance.

The Perils of Managed Care

Some of the concerns of the critics of managed care which should be brought to board members' attention include:

- Mental health outcomes for the poor appear to be worse in a managed care environment than in fee-for-service, according to recent studies.
- Capitated payments provide incentives to limit, reduce or withhold services. In fact, despite the rush to contain costs and move

the child to a less restrictive and less costly alternative, the client may not be ready, thus adversely affecting the anticipated outcome.

- The behavior of seriously emotionally disturbed children who have suffered both poverty and abuse is not susceptible to quick fixes, in managed care or in any other system. Demanding substantial savings in the short-term would do damage to both the clinical and financial expectations.
- Medication is a problematic area. Newly-developed drugs are often very expensive, and MCOs have formularies which usually do not include these costly items. Drug substitutions are effective as a cost containment strategy, but they may not always be effective in the behavior modification of children.
- The chronically mentally ill may be short-changed in an MCO since this population is in need of long term care.
- Persons with chronic mental illness tend to have a high dropout rate. There will be little incentive in a capitation arrangement for staff to aggressively follow-up missed appointments.

In fact, in the past, the chronically mentally ill were specifically *excluded* from HMO coverage through such contract clauses as *conditions which are chronic or not likely to respond to short-term treatment.* Unless providers have a capitation payment which is adjusted for high risk or heavy utilization, resources will not be adequate and care will suffer or be severely rationed. The state, which sets the Medicaid monthly rate, expects to realize savings under managed care compared with the fee-for-service system. Typically, these savings range from 5 to 10 percent and are included in the calculations of the rate. The fee-for-service calculations are based on State Medicaid fee schedules, which, for practitioners, have been historically low:

> The uninsured, for whom nonprofit providers of care have been a traditional safety net, will impose an inordinate financial burden on children's services agencies. Managed care has achieved savings by negotiating discounts from providers in exchange for inclusion in the MCO networks. Moreover, the federal government continues to shrink existing health and welfare programs. And shifting the poor uninsured to state psychiatric facilities

becomes more difficult as most states are winding down these hospitals.

Relief is not in sight except for expansion of child health insurance programs for low-income children. This new program, State Children's Health Insurance Program (S-CHIP) provides funds to states for the initiation and expansion of child health services to uninsured, low-income children, in accordance with the provisions of a new Title XXI of the Social Security Act. States will have the option of using new matching federal funds to expand Medicaid, or develop or expand existing separate child health insurance programs. Whether or not mental health services for children are included, and how much, will depend on the individual state programs or their corresponding State Medicaid programs. In New York, for example, in the past, the program for low-income and uninsured children, Child Health Plus, did not cover inpatient mental health services, but did cover 20 clinic visits per year for mental health care, and another 40 visits were available annually for alcohol and substance abuse treatment. With the availability of federal funding, New York will be enrolling more children, and expanding services. Eligibility has been changed to include children in families whose gross household income is less than 230 percent of the federal poverty level. Benefits have been expanded to cover inpatient mental health, alcohol and substance abuse services, over-the-counter drugs, dental, vision, speech and hearing services. Medicaid eligibility was also expanded to include children in families with net household income up to 133 percent of the federal poverty level.

The Continuing Education of Board Members

Longstanding board members should not be permitted to stagnate, and new board members should be oriented to the agency's mission and activities, and the environment in which it operates. Because of the volatile nature of the health and human services field, board members have to keep abreast by enlarging their understanding and participating in formal educational activities of the board. The board as a whole is obligated to stimulate and assist each other, especially those with special expertise or skill in a needed field. But it is the chairperson or board president who carries the greatest obligation to assure ongoing education and training. While that person may be thought of as a fellow student, the leadership for such activities should emanate from the chair.

The executive director also plays an important role in the continuing education of board members by keeping members informed of the work of the agency, and significant events or movements which affect the agency. Regular reports by the executive at board meetings, and the creation of special task forces to focus on specific issues not covered by standing committees can be helpful to the board as a whole. While statistics and generalities are important in making presentations, such as the number of new managed care contracts, or the impact on revenues, it is important to personalize the information with typical cases. Being mindful of client confidentiality, cases could be described demonstrating easier access to care, better continuity of care or family bonding, or stability after crisis intervention. Failures are as important to report as successes, and whether managed care did or could make a difference. The everyday drama of the staff's work should be shared with the board, which should not be condemned exclusively to the review of dry numbers and abstract issues.

As more and more children's services agencies become involved with managed care, an individual case could be presented at selected meetings of the board on how clinical care was affected, if at all; how financing and cash flow has changed for the individual case, by program, and for the agency as a whole.

How detailed should a board member's knowledge be about the world of managed care? Certainly, board members should never micromanage the organization, nor do they need to know the technical details about how to distinguish between average costs and marginal costs. But they do need to understand the concepts behind these definitions, the importance of the distinction, and how that relates to financial viability.

Similarly, board members need not know how to purchase stop-loss insurance, or how to define it (a form of reinsurance purchased by a health plan to protect itself from excessive expenditures incurred in the fulfillment of its contractual benefits), but they should understand the need to protect the agency from the atypically expensive care of individuals.

Board members need not know how to co-mingle operating revenues, but they should understand the concept or desirability of merging funding streams so as to afford staff the greatest flexibility in the management of the organization.

Board members need not know how to develop risk-adjusted rates. But because of its importance in the care of SED individuals in a capitated environment, they need to understand the assumption of financial risk when the art of rate-adjustment for psychiatric disorders is still so rudimentary. Neither the federal government, nor any state or academic center has been able to develop psychiatric Diagnosis-Related Groups (DRGs) which have a significant correlation with resource utilization.

Board members need not know how the numbers for the *carve-out* (removal of the services and populations with especially high costs from the mainstream health plan) were determined, but they need to know that their agency is treating a high-cost population by the behavioral health specialists who can most effectively treat this population. They also need to know that this arrangement could be one step in the direction of a fully-capitated plan by a mainstream MCO, or a permanent solution to the care of a high-risk population.

Board members need to understand that an agency's success at managing care depends to a great degree on how much of the care continuum the agency itself provides and manages, without having to know what should be done in-house, and what should be referred out.

CONCLUSIONS

Like it or not, nonprofit children's services agencies will be engaging the world of managed care in the forthcoming years. Whether it be on a full-capitation, partial-capitation, or discounted fee-for-service basis, whether it be for child welfare or behavioral health, or both, whether it be for the short-term or the long haul, life will not be the same again. The world of risk will become a sharp reality.

Such agencies, on the other hand, will have the opportunity to offer mainstream MCOs what they need, expertise from specialists for a high-cost population, at prices significantly lower in a community setting than in costly acute care hospitals.

These agencies' abilities to fulfill their mission to serve the uninsured will be severely taxed, as discounted rates and the tightening of government welfare and health programs cut off sources of cross subsidies. The only bright light on the horizon will be the expansion of child health insurance programs.

Small agencies without multiple sources of funding, or those lacking capability or the will to move ahead quickly, will be unable to assume risk in this competitive environment, and will become the object of acquisitions (or mergers) by the larger agencies.

RECOMMENDATIONS

Agencies will have to streamline their organizations by eliminating redundancies and inefficiencies, developing the most efficient mix of human resources, focusing on the most cost-effective treatment modalities, and ascertaining their average and marginal costs in order to remain financially viable in a competitive market.

Boards of directors need to become conversant with the philosophy and economics of managed care if they are to effectively serve the agency. Education and training in the volatile fields of welfare and behavioral health need to be ongoing. Information imparted in May may be stale in December. The board president, the administrator and key staff need to work together to assure that information and significant events are shared on an ongoing basis.

Members should be appointed to the board who have some background and experience with managed care and special needs populations.

Research needs to continue to develop and apply the tools for risk assessment and risk adjustment for high-risk users so that plans and providers will be adequately compensated.

Even with adherence to the above recommendations, there is no way of telling whether specialty plans are here to stay, or whether, given the appropriate financial incentives, mainstream MCOs will take on the high-risk patients they currently shun. Market unpredictability is a significant aspect of risk. Are board members prepared for the challenge?

REFERENCES

Cain, D. (1991). *Board Talk with Dan Cain*. The Cain Consulting Group: Hawarden, IA, Tape 1.

Currents, Medicaid Managed Care (1997, Summer). New York: United Hospital Fund V. 2, Number 2, 3-5.

Data Bulletin. (1997). Washington, DC: Center for Studying Health System Change, 6.

Freudenheim, M. (1997, November 27). Baby Boomers Force New Rules for HMOs. *The New York Times*, A1, D2.

Houle, C. O. (1989), *Governing Boards*. San Francisco: Jossey-Bass Publishers. 51-54.

Howe, F. (1995). *Welcome to the Board, Your Guide to Effective Participation.* San Francisco: Jossey-Bass Publishers. 13-14, 24.

Hutchins, J. (1997, Fall). Managing Managed Care for Families. *Children's Voice,* 28-29.

Issue Brief. (1997, May). Health Plans and Providers: Shifting Roles. Washington, DC: Center for Studying Health System Change Number 9, 3.

Risk Adjustment, A Key to Changing Incentives in the Health Insurance Market (1997, March). Washington, DC: The Alpha Center.

Schlesinger, M. (1986). On the Limits of Expanding Health Care Reform: Chronic Care in Prepaid Settings. *The Milbank Quarterly,* Vol. 64, No. 2, 189-215.

State Initiatives in Health Care Reform (1997, April). Carve-Out Arrangements in Managed Care: Experience Suggests Value Despite Questions About Long-term Viability. Washington, DC: The Alpha Center. 8-9.

Zuckerman, S., Evans A., and Holahan J. (1997, August). Questions for States as They Turn to Medicaid Managed Care. *New Federalism Issues and Options for States.* Washington, DC: The Urban Institute. Series A, No. A-11.

Alternative Board Structures
to Accommodate New Demands

L. D. Williams, MSW, ACSW

SUMMARY. The nonprofit governance revolution is going beyond the back-to-basics approach and is charting new governance territory for today's progressive and successful organization. New concepts are gently combined with time-tested basics to form a more dynamic and productive approach. The tremendously positive results are just beginning to be realized. Core components of progressive alternative board structures include: (1) the CEO has a significant place providing support, help, and goodwill to the board of directors; (2) there is a concerted effort to clearly define the different roles and functions that differentiate board and staff efforts; (3) the successful organization continually assesses and responds to incessant change in the business environment; and (4) nonprofit agencies of today are developing new organizational and board structures that accommodate vision, action, and achievement.

The true measure of the strength of a nonprofit organization lies in its ability to adapt to changes that occur in its environment. Most of the time when change occurs, the last part of the organization that experiences improvement through change is the board of directors. In today's nonprofit world, we must have open minds and truly assess new ways of doing business so we may meet the new demands we face. *[Article copies available for a fee from The Haworth Document Delivery Service: 1-800-342-9678. E-mail address: getinfo@haworthpressinc.com <Website: http://www.haworth pressinc.com>]*

KEYWORDS. Nonprofits, boards, structures, CEOs, management

[Haworth co-indexing entry note]: "Alternative Board Structures to Accommodate New Demands." Williams, L. D. Co-published simultaneously in *Residential Treatment for Children & Youth* (The Haworth Press, Inc.) Vol. 16, No. 4, 1999, pp. 63-76; and: *The New Board: Changing Issues, Roles and Relationships* (ed: Nadia Ehrlich Finkelstein, and Raymond Schimmer) The Haworth Press, Inc., 1999, pp. 63-76. Single or multiple copies of this article are available for a fee from The Haworth Document Delivery Service [1-800-342-9678, 9:00 a.m. - 5:00 p.m. (EST). E-mail address: getinfo@haworthpressinc.com].

63

The nonprofit corporate world is extraordinarily complex when compared to the normal business corporate world. Nonprofit organizations depend a great deal on unpaid volunteers, usually are intertwined into the fabric of the community, and often defy the reality of the generally accepted truism, "without money your business will go bankrupt." Staff of the nonprofit are at times inadequately paid and indifferently governed. Yet, in spite of this, the organization continues to serve the community, and in some instances, registers significant improvement in its services and activities year after year.

Nonprofit organizations are complex. Yet, there are some identifiable commonalities. These include the following:

- The relationship and partnership of the CEO and the board is crucial. The primary staff leader is important to the board because it must have executive support, help, and goodwill to be successful in its governance function. Roles of the CEO and the board must be clearly defined with identification as to "who does what best."
- Nonprofit boards are composed of non-compensated volunteers whose sole purpose in serving is to help those in the community who hurt and/or need help. The level of board involvement in daily operations should generally be nil. There are important reasons for the board to be careful not to overstep its role. Boards should work to become better at what they should be doing.
- The final two points that play a part in defining board structure are role and function of staff and identification of what may well be the ultimate alternative board structure for the large, progressive, successful nonprofit organization.

NEW DEMANDS, AND THE NECESSITY OF VISION AND CHANGE

Tom Peters and Nancy Austin, in *A Passion for Excellence* (1985), write,

So a revolution is brewing. What kind of revolution? In large measure it is, in fact, a 'back to basics' revolution. The management systems, schemes, devices, and structures promoted during the last quarter century have added up to distractions from the main ideas: the achievement of sustainable growth and equity. (p. xvii)

Peters and Austin certainly identified the management theme of the eighties, "Back to Basics," and correctly characterized it as a revolution. On the eve of the twenty-first century, there is a new revolution that began a few years ago and continues to gain disciples: the nonprofit governance revolution. In every way, it is very different from the management revolution of the eighties and nineties. Instead of going back to the basics, this revolution is charting new governance territory for nonprofit organizations. New concepts are gently combined with time-tested basics to form a more dynamic and productive approach to governance. The tremendously positive results are just beginning to be realized.

The demands on today's nonprofit organization are many and varied. There are constant concerns about mission, financing of operations and programs, performance of boards of directors, appropriate level of governance, competent executive leadership, professionally credentialed staff, etc. Additionally, every organization has its problems and challenges. Often, the question is "Should we improve what we have, or should we create something new?" In his book, *Mission Possible* (1997), Ken Blanchard has a unique answer to this dilemma: "Which approach is better–improving what is, or creating what isn't? ANSWER? YES!" (p. xxi).

Organizational problems become more complex as the organization responds to societal change. In every nonprofit organization, there is no greater problem than a malfunctioning board of directors. If governance fails, the potential for success drops significantly. The governance problem is more fully understood when one realizes most board members do not have the time to think, search, read and prepare concepts for the future of the nonprofit. They may instead become entangled in matters of little or no importance and fall into the trap of complete ineffectiveness. The situation cries for resolution and solution.

During the past twenty years, the rules have changed substantially in philanthropic and other nonprofit organizations. Nonprofit organizations suddenly find the private, for-profit sector competing in their arena because funds have been made available to support and pay for many services. For-profit businesses move in and try to move the nonprofit agencies out. However, the nonprofit sector has an advantage in that it can effectively recruit volunteers who serve as unpaid workers in the organization and develop fundraising activities that appeal to the philanthropy of others. The spirit of volunteerism and the spirit of philanthropy that have been hallmarks of our American society, openly and proudly displayed by our nation's nonprofit sector, are alive and well. Myriad people volunteer to serve more causes than ever before. More money is donated to more causes today than at any time in the past. There are those in our society who embrace the thought that volunteerism and philanthropy help form the backbone of our national character and purpose. Our volunteers of today exhibit caring, compassion, concern, and commitment that is unparalleled. They have brought us to a high level of sophistication in much of the nonprofit sector, and they have produced a direct challenge to the best in the for-profit business world. Nonprofit organizations are developing new organizational and board structures that accommodate vision, action, and achievement. The visionary nonprofit agencies of today are vibrant, well-run organizations that accomplish much on behalf of others. However, there is a need for constant introspection to single out what is required for the organization to remain productive and true to its mission.

The hallmark of a successful organization today is its ability to continually assess and respond to continuous, ongoing change in the business environment. This is especially true of the human service organization. The needs (problems) of clients shift; government (politics) realigns its priorities; the mood of the public becomes uneasy and demanding; competition becomes a major, threatening force; historical funding resources dry up; regulations become more stringent and punitive. As these and other changes occur, innovative organizations adjust, transform, revamp, adapt, and/or take new direction. In a word, they innovate. Creativity becomes the norm and not the exception. Therefore, how an organization responds to the daily pressures that it confronts will determine whether it is destined to succeed or fail. To a large extent, the board of directors plays a major role in such success or failure.

Where does one start in trying to position an organization "to become all that it can be?" Of course, success begins with the governing body, the chief executive officer, and the staff assembled by the

CEO. James P. Collins and Jerry I. Porras in *Built to Last* (1994) declare that great organizations are led by:

> . . . clock builders, not time tellers . . . Visionary companies do not ask, What should we value? They ask, What do we actually value deep down to our toes? . . . The builders of visionary companies seek alignment in strategies, in tactics, in organization systems, in structure, in incentive systems, in building layout, in job design–in everything. (p. 7)

> . . . Intentions are all fine and good, but it is the translation of those intentions into concrete items–mechanisms with teeth–that can make the difference between becoming a visionary company or forever remaining a wannabe. (p. 8)

One of the keys to resounding success in a nonprofit organization is the level of ability and skills exhibited by the CEO and a close relationship developed between management and the board of directors. Management of a human service agency is too often placed in the hands of an executive who is not capable, who depends on the board of directors to make most, if not all, decisions. The lack of leadership from the executive can cause a virtual vacuum where creativity and vision cannot develop. Amateurism in management is inexcusable except for the neophyte; boards are foolish to place agency leadership in the hands of an untested and untried person unless opportunities and assistance in learning the art of management are provided.

One of the major tasks of the chief executive is to convert purpose into performance. Boards should require the executive to be accountable, always acting within the parameters of the board's clearly defined ethics, values, and established limits. John Carver, in his book *Boards That Make a Difference* (1996), says:

> The skills sought in a CEO are not those associated with responsibility, but with accountability. For example, grant writing, plant maintenance, and accounting are not the point. Executive job design, leadership, strategic organization, and setting a climate of creative achievement are . . . The chief executive officer is accountable to the board of directors for (1) achievement of ends policy and (2) non-violation of executive limitations policies. (p. 107-108)

In other words, it is important that the board of directors spend its time creating, visioning, and monitoring, while the executive acts to achieve the goals set by the board. The board does not question or prescribe methods of goal achievement. It simply identifies goals and requires clearly identified outcomes.

If an organization is to be successful, it must get beyond asking who are we, and who do we want to become? The questions must be: What are our core values and central purpose for existence? What is the best way for us to define our intentions, agree on the appropriate action, and move to set in motion forces that will produce the desired outcome?

If there is one word that can be used to describe the key to success in any business (profit or nonprofit), it is ACTION. While vision and planning are an integral part of an organization's success, the time always comes when plans must be implemented. If one does not "do it," it is impossible to know if "it" will be successful, if improvements can be made, if adjustments are indicated, or if "it" is just a bad idea.

Another danger is that analysis of a proposed project/activity/program may be carried on too long, and ACTION is impeded. Stick to the basics and don't worry about achieving perfection before implementing the project. It is generally better to analyze the project in progress than it is to overanalyze the plans. It is incumbent on every organization to take advantage of every opportunity if there is to be progress through positive response to the business environment.

The importance of maximizing opportunities cannot be overemphasized. In the mid-sixties, Peter Drucker said, in *Managing for Results* (1964):

> Maximizing opportunities shows how to move the business from yesterday to today–thereby making it ready for the new challenges of tomorrow. It shows the existing activities that should be pushed and those that should be abandoned. And it brings out the new things that might multiply results in the market or in the company's field of knowledge. Maximizing resources, finally, is the step from insight to action. It establishes priorities. And by concentrating resources on priorities it ensures that energy and efforts go to work where performance can produce the greatest results. (p. 140-141)

Thomas J. Peters and Robert H. Waterman, in their book, *In Search of Excellence* (1982), identified a worthy axiom in their study of this country's most successful companies, "Do It; Fix It; Try It." They characterize this slogan as "a bias for action, for getting on with it" (p. 13). This is an absolutely crucial principle if one is to be highly successful in human services. In organizations where this axiom is practiced, innovation is not an option, it is a requirement.

The complex environment in which organizations operate often leads to making the "complex" more complex. This is befuddling at best and destructive at worst. When an organization's structure, activities, and services are kept simple, understanding is enhanced, basics are emphasized, implementation is easier. The reward for simplicity is evident in staff support, client understanding, and community response. People have a need to understand. Reduce everything in the organization to its least common denominator. Complexity leads to the intellect overpowering wisdom and ultimately to confusion. We must all learn to keep it simple. This includes board, staff, and organizational structure.

A key element to organizational health and prosperity is a vision of where the organization can go, what it can do, and when. There are organizations that have existed for one hundred years or more without ever developing or utilizing a vision. They take care of business as it arises, are reactive to forces that confront them, and seldom take risks. However, no human service organization ever became all it could be (or a leading force) without a powerful vision or a willingness to take prudent risks to achieve its vision. The vision may originate with the board of directors, the CEO, members of the staff, clients or from the organization's constituency.

A vision seldom comes to fruition in its original form. The vision ages, expands, contracts, and develops as the organization's players understand and buy into the articulation of the vision. As the vision develops, a determination is made regarding the risks that must be taken. The mission of the organization is carefully considered in light of the vision. The visions of tomorrow prepare us for the future, but they honor the present and always remember the past. One should always remember that no vision is too wild or impossible to reach. If it serves the central theme of the organization, if resources are available or can be developed, if the players in the organization are willing to work hard to make it happen, it can be done. Within these parameters, some adjustments may need to be made to the vision, but it can work.

COMPARATIVE MODELS OF BOARD STRUCTURE

Three board structure models commonly used in nonprofit organizations today are:

- The traditional model, in which the board insists on ultimate control of every aspect of the organization's function.
- The corporate model, in which the board allows all operational control to rest with the chief executive officer.
- The multi-corporation model, which allows the chief executive officer to run the organization with only minimum board-approved goals, minimum general guidance, and constant monitoring of results.

Other board models exist, but the three listed above or variations of them are most often used in today's nonprofit agencies. When a board chooses a model that would best meet an organization's needs, it should consider a number of factors:

- The traditional model would be best for the organization with a small number of programs, small staff, lack of sophistication in methods and program, and if the chief executive officer is neither experienced and/or a strong, knowledgeable leader. However, even under these circumstances, it behooves boards to chart a course that will eventually lead to the relinquishment of control of method and focus on required outcomes only. This may require providing management learning opportunities for the executive, and understanding that growth and skill development take time. One of the clear dangers in this model is that the board will spend valuable time revisiting, reexamining, redoing, and rehashing what the executive and/or staff have already done.
- The corporate model of governance requires the board to exercise discipline that helps it focus on goals rather than methods. This board does not demand approval authority over the minuscule matters but leaves the organization's day-to-day operation in the hands of a trusted, knowledgeable leader, the CEO, and

works very hard to differentiate between the small and large issues that confront the organization. It does not allow itself to become entangled in matters of little importance. Always working to get better at its jobs, this board tries to determine which matters require its time and energy, and how it can become better at the work it should be doing.

- The multiple-corporation organizational model is at once the most complex and the most simple of models. It is the most complex in that there are multiple corporations, each of which has corporate components (articles of incorporation, bylaws, financial activities, boards of directors, etc.). It is the simplest model in that the blending of most services and legal functions can be carried out cooperatively, thereby producing economies of scale and function.

It is, of course, possible for a board to create its own unique model by drawing on parts derived from the models described above.

THE MULTIPLE CORPORATION MODEL: ONE EXAMPLE

The structure is relatively simple:

- The Parent Corporation becomes a management company existing for the purpose of providing management and other services to its corporate affiliates in support of their 501 (c) 3 charitable organization missions.
- The Parent Corporation's board of directors is composed of:
  1. The chairman of each affiliate corporation.
  2. Seven additional at-large members elected by the board of the Parent Corporation.
  3. The President/CEO of the Parent Corporation.

An agreement is signed between the Parent Corporation and each of its affiliates. This is an agreement that is irrevocable for a term of 20 years; upon expiration of the original agreement, an additional 20-year term automatically kicks in unless the Parent Corporation elects to cancel the agreement.

- Contracts, memoranda of understanding, and lease agreements are executed to formalize the business relationship between the Parent Corporation and its affiliates.

- Services provided by the Parent Corporation include:

  a. Administrative support and management training services including consultation, services of the president, and services of other Parent Corporation personnel.
  b. Complete bookkeeping, accounting and business services including all banking, debt service, checking services, lines of credit, etc.
  c. Human Resource services including leased employees for all affiliates, employee benefits administration, employee file maintenance service, recruiting services, employee orientation services, professional liability insurance.
  d. Complete funding of operations for the foundation affiliate.
  e. Services of foundation to all affiliates for funds development, public and community relations, advertising, marketing, publications.
  f. Transcription services through a central dictation system.
  g. Telephone and front desk reception services for all affiliates.
  h. Support staff intervention team to address periodic support needs for all affiliates.

- Parent Corporation policies are formulated to guide affiliates in required philosophies, role expectations, corporate objectives, required procedural matters, financial policies, corporate relations, etc.
- The Parent Corporation board of directors performs the following functions:

  a. Hires, evaluates, and terminates the Parent Corporation CEO.
  b. Exercises debt approval and controls debt for all affiliates.
  c. Appoints a nominating committee and approves the appointment of all affiliate board members.
  d. Exercises its authority to move funds around within the affiliate corporate structure to address deficits, purchases, income and expense needs.
  e. Authorizes the CEO of the Parent Corporation to hire, evaluate, terminate all employees of all corporations.
  f. Authorizes the Parent Corporation CEO to hire, supervise, evaluate, and terminate all executives of all affiliates and to act as CEO for all affiliates.

In the opinion of this author, the Multiple Corporation Board Structure Model has many advantages; however, this structure should only be adopted if the appropriate groundwork has been laid. Before proceeding to adopt such a structure, a complete organizational assessment is essential. The intent to develop this model should then become part of the organization's strategic plan. A lot of time for board brainstorming as to what it wants to achieve, how the new structure will be different from the previous one, concerns, etc., is necessary, yet, beware of the "nay sayers" who will want to impede or stop progress.

The Multiple Corporation Board Structure offers the following advantages:

1. Organizations with large, diverse programs that have little in common will be able to see programs prosper under the new structure. For example, before establishing separate corporations, an organization might have a Family Service Division, a Mental Health Division, a Children's Residential Treatment Division, a Child Abuse and Neglect Division, and a Boys & Girls Club Division. All these divisions could be combined into the following sectors, each with a separate board of directors and a separate executive: Family Service Division and Mental Health Division may be combined to become Family Service Agency Inc. (or Mental Health Agency Inc.); Children's Residential Treatment Division could become Children's Residential Treatment Agency Inc.; Child Abuse and Neglect Division could become Child Abuse and Neglect Agency Inc.; and Boys & Girls Club Division could become Boys & Girls Club Inc. The Parent Corporation might be one of the existing agencies or a completely separate entity. The Parent Corporation then might found a 509 (a) Charitable Foundation Inc., and an Asset Management Agency Inc.

When this hypothetical reorganization is completed, the above organization would have a Parent Corporation, four human service agencies (or three if one of the agencies is the Parent Corp.), a charitable foundation, and an asset management agency. The Parent Corporation board would be the most powerful board of directors, and there would be six (or five) additional boards of directors. In the past, the organization may have had one board of directors with 30 to 35 board members. With the reorganization, there may be as many as 100 board members in six or seven nonprofit corporations. This allows the boards of directors to concentrate only on their agency's programs. The four human service agency boards would concentrate only on their agency vision, mission, and their overall governance efforts. Their facilities, equipment, automobiles, etc., are all provided and maintained by the Asset Management Agency. Their resource development, marketing, public relations, publications, etc., are all provided by the Charitable Foundation. A review of the previously listed Parent Corporation activities will remind us that many support services are available outside to each of the agencies, yet all of them function under the same organizational umbrella.

2. Financial information will be easier to follow with fewer cost centers in any one agency.
3. General and Administrative (G&A) costs for any of the agencies will be less because much of these are covered under a purchase of service agreement with the Parent Corporation. Another advantage is that G&A costs which are usually non-allowable, are allowable in contracts as a purchase of service.
4. A problem in any one of the corporation's affiliates impacts only that affiliate. Each one stands alone as a separate corporation responsible for solving its problems. While the Parent Corporation has a vested interest in assisting, the Parent Corporation does not own the problems. However, there will be other executives and other boards willing to assist in problem solving, if requested. The Parent Corporation is always there to step in and fill an immediate need while the affiliate is working on resolution.
5. Affiliates are required to purchase needed services first from the Parent Corporation or from another affiliate. If the needed service is not available through one of the organization's companies, they are then permitted to go outside to fulfill the need for goods or services.
6. Board size can be kept to a reasonable number depending on the services and needs of each agency. The size may vary between seven and twenty board members (or choose any other number that can be adequately supported).
7. Each board can have fewer standing committees. Some of the agencies might function with only three standing committees:

Planning/Resource Committee, Assessment/Evaluation Committee, Executive Committee. Any other board committees could be ad hoc (time limited and/or task specific).

8. With management (executives of affiliate agencies) being overseen by the President/CEO of the Parent Corporation (including recruiting, hiring, monitoring, disciplining, evaluating, and terminating), the boards can now spend their time in visioning, planning, monitoring, fundraising, community relations, and become better at what they should be doing.

9. Other agencies in the community can now consider affiliating with the Parent Corporation because they would have the best of all worlds: they can maintain their identities and, within parameters, their independence, while having the support and backing of a large, well-run organization.

10. When put together, the major assets (buildings, equipment, endowments) of the organization can be protected from litigation. This will vary from state to state, and an organization should engage a good corporate attorney for advice on the appropriate structure.

In summary, the above model is really a simple structure. All affiliates are independent within the limits of the mission and basic corporate policy of the Parent Corporation. There are a few controls previously listed that the Parent Corporation maintains in order to assure continuity and quality of effort. Additionally, affiliate bylaws cannot be changed without the approval of the Parent Corporation board.

As one looks at the times and assesses what needs to be done to improve our charitable nonprofit organizations, the need for some overhaul of the structure and function of many boards of directors becomes apparent. The Multiple Corporation Board Structure as presented in this paper actually mirrors the organizational structure of a human service organization that reorganized eleven years ago. This organization ended 1986 with $2.4 million in income and expenses. The 1997 audited year-end financial statement shows $20 million in income and expenses. This growth of more than 800% in eleven years is directly attributable to the reorganization into multiple corporations, restructuring the board of directors to match the reorganization, and the application of advanced management principles.

The true measure of the strength of a nonprofit organization lies in its ability to adapt to changes that occur in its environment. Most of the time when change occurs, the last part of the organization that experiences improvement through change is the board of directors. In most nonprofit organizations throughout the country, it would be a giant step forward if the board of directors considered alternative board structures to accommodate new demands. The new demands are coming fast and furiously, and we must assess ways to meet them. Nonprofit boards of directors must therefore search for new ways to do business. Only then will their organizations become all they can be.

REFERENCES

Blanchard, Ken. (1997) *Mission Possible*. New York: McGraw-Hill.

Carver, John. (1990) *Boards That Make a Difference*. San Francisco: Jossey-Bass.

Collins, James C. and Jerry I. Porras. (1994, 1997) *Built to Last: Successful Habits of Visionary Companies*. New York: HarperCollins Publishers.

Drucker, Peter F. (1964) *Managing for Results*. New York: Harper & Row.

Peters, Tom and Nancy Austin. (1985) *A Passion for Excellence: The Leadership Difference*. New York: Warner Books.

Peters, Tom and Robert H. Waterman. (1982) *In Search of Excellence*. New York: Harper & Row.

The Board Change Process:
One Agency's Experience

Nadia Ehrlich Finkelstein, MS, ACSW
Raymond Schimmer, MAT

SUMMARY. Boards of Directors have ample reason to reconsider the fundamental structures and methods of operation during periods of fluidity and change. The authors present the experience of one children and family services agency's Board of Directors as the Board analyzed and restructured itself. They discuss the context of the Board's decision to proceed, the organization of a task force, the collection of data on current and best practice, and the formulation of recommendations. The changes made to Board structure are listed, and a preliminary report on their impact to date, along with plans for future reassessment, are described. *[Article copies available for a fee from The Haworth Document Delivery Service: 1-800-342-9678. E-mail address: getinfo@haworthpress inc.com <Website: http://www.haworthpressinc.com>]*

KEYWORDS. Nonprofits, boards, treatment centers, management, change

It was not the best of times, but it certainly was not the worst of times, either. Indeed, by many measurements, when the Center's Board of Directors gathered for its Annual Retreat in October 1995, times were rather good. The Center had all the serious problems that nonprofit multiservice treatment agencies face at the end of the twen-

[Haworth co-indexing entry note]: "The Board Change Process: One Agency's Experience." Finkelstein, Nadia Ehrlich, and Raymond Schimmer. Co-published simultaneously in *Residential Treatment for Children & Youth* (The Haworth Press, Inc.) Vol. 16, No. 4, 1999, pp. 77-90; and: *The New Board: Changing Issues, Roles and Relationships* (ed: Nadia Ehrlich Finkelstein, and Raymond Schimmer) The Haworth Press, Inc., 1999, pp. 77-90. Single or multiple copies of this article are available for a fee from The Haworth Document Delivery Service [1-800-342-9678, 9:00 a.m. - 5:00 p.m. (EST). E-mail address: getinfo@haworthpressinc.com].

77

tieth century, but its Board was not confronting desperate and compelling circumstance on the Friday evening of Retreat Weekend.

Taylor, Chait, and Holland (1996, p. 46), in "The New Work of the Nonprofit Board," commented on what they believe to be the typical board posture in such a situation:

> A sympathetic explanation for the reluctance of most boards to experiment with substantial governance reforms would be the trustees' desire to do no harm. A less charitable explanation would be the trustees' desire to do no work.

And yet, before the Board members left for home on Saturday evening, they had determined to review–and to change–the entirety of the Board's foundation in the year to come.

Three months later, at a regular meeting of the Board, the Vice President recounted the desires expressed by his colleagues during the Retreat: Director participation in Center business should be more substantive and productive; the Board should be able to secure the skills and support of more community members without necessarily enlarging itself; the Board should look directly at its role in raising money; and most importantly, the *Bylaws* and *Policies and Procedures* should be revised so that the desired changes would become part of the Board's foundation.

This was certainly not the charge of a group trying "to do no work." How, then, did the Board come to such a point without the impetus of serious crisis?

Many conditions favored change. First, there was opportunity. Four months before the Retreat, the Board had installed a new Board President and had hired a new Executive Director. The sense of "fresh start" was almost palpable. Next, the Board's recent search for the executive director, while taxing, had been invigorating. The Board members, particularly those who had been on the Search Committee, felt that they had worked together effectively on a matter of serious consequence, and felt that their potential could–and *should*–be tapped again.

There was also necessity, which Board members perceived even though it did not manifest itself as an imminent crisis of great moment. The region's economics were changing. Seasoned executives, long the mainstays of the area's nonprofit boards, were being transferred, downsized, or given much larger job descriptions as their companies merged or were taken over. Younger executives were struggling with employment uncertainty while trying to raise their own families. Demographic trends were unfolding: "old line" board members began reducing community activity as they entered retirement. Clearly, the Center needed to study the personal circumstances and experiences of its Directors, and to modify Board life to fit new conditions.

The Center had also grown vastly more complex since the existing structure had been defined. The *Bylaws* had gone through twelve partial revisions over two decades without ever being completely rewritten. Exigencies of the past that once shaped policy had receded like ancient glaciers, leaving behind a rubble of incongruous provisions and guidelines that were incomprehensible to contemporary directors. The Center itself had grown 2-1/2 times in ten years; its old governance structure creaked as the Board sought to maintain informed oversight.

Finally, those Directors at the Retreat recognized the challenges faced by many treatment centers at the end of the twentieth century: managed care, industry consolidation, rapidly changing service needs and technology, the rise of the for-profit agency, and increasing demands for the time and attention of those who traditionally had served to direct nonprofit treatment centers. The Center needed the participation of its Directors more than ever, but to secure that, it would have to accommodate them. The Center would have to use the Directors' limited time more efficiently, recognize that few, if any, of them could work intensively on every aspect of Center activity, and figure out how to share power without compromising direction.

At the December Board meeting following the Retreat, a blue ribbon Board Restructuring Task Force was established to study the issues.

TASK FORCE CHARGE

The charge by the Board to the Task Force was to examine the current Board structure and method of operation and to propose recommendations for change as appropriate to deal with the challenges of the next decade. These recommendations were to be submitted to the May 1996 meeting of the Board of Directors for discussion. The

Board would then vote to accept or reject any or all of the recommendations at the following meeting in June.

TASK FORCE COMPOSITION

The Task Force was composed of ten members, including six current Directors, one of whom was the President, three who were former Board members, and one recently retired member of the executive staff of the agency. The Task Force was staffed by the Executive Director, who chaired the meetings, and by the Executive Assistant. All meetings were open to any member of the Board who wanted to attend.

TASK FORCE WORK PLAN

The Task Force met eight times over a four-month period and engaged in a series of tasks to accomplish the following objectives:

1. Identify principal tasks likely to face the Board in the next decade.
2. Review current Board architecture and operating guidelines including Board composition, *Bylaws, Policies and Procedures.*
3. Prepare recommendations concerning the Board structure and policies that would enable the Board to more easily manage the anticipated future challenges.

METHOD

Task Force composition was key to the efficient operation and charge accomplishment in a very limited amount of time. Most, though not all, group members knew each other. Several had worked together previously, and came together already possessing a great deal of mutual respect. Nevertheless, the group was sufficiently diverse to allow for multiple questions and perspectives. After some initial discussion concerning the reasons for the project, the group took ownership of the charge given to it by the Board. This allowed it to focus immediately on the development and implementation of a work plan.

First, the Task Force asked the Center librarian to conduct a computer search of pertinent literature, which resulted in the distribution of articles to all of the Task Force members (see References). The articles were eventually summarized by individual committee members and presented for discussion. The process was stimulating and established something of a common knowledge base among the Task Force members.

The next job was to develop a set of shared values, or desired outcomes, that would guide all further deliberations. Through the technique commonly known as "brainstorming," the group identified 21 characteristics that an efficient Board would require. The list was then screened for redundancy and reduced to 9 (see Appendix A).

In preparation for recommendations on the revision of *Bylaws*, the Task Force established a *Bylaws* subcommittee, whose members conducted a comprehensive review of the current *Bylaws*, including a separate but related document known as *Policies and Procedures*. *Policies and Procedures* had been intended originally to provide detail about the implementation of various aspects of the *Bylaws*; however, in the course of this review, it became apparent that it was often difficult to determine which material belonged in the *Bylaws*, and which should be in *Policies and Procedures*.

The group also chose to develop a "Current and Best Practice Questionnaire." Two subcommittees were then established–one the "Current Practice" subcommittee, and the other the "Best Practice" subcommittee–to accomplish this task. These subcommittees intended to use the Questionnaire to describe the Center's own internal practice, and then to use it again in discussions with six agencies known nationally for innovative approaches in the area of board functioning. The agencies selected have gained their colleagues' respect for sound operation, creativity, and willingness to change. The actual selection was based on specific recommendations by the Task Force members familiar with the field, and by consulting with colleagues in other organizations. The Task Force recognized that there are many more organizations than the six chosen who are doing exemplary work, but was constrained by time to do a limited survey.

The Center's Executive Director was charged to ask the Executives of the six "Best Practice" organizations if they would share their Board documents and participate in a telephone interview with a Task Force member. The Executives responded generously. Individual agencies were assigned to Task Force members for follow-up. A copy of the "Current and Best Practice Questionnaire" was then mailed to the CEO interviewees prior to the telephone conference. The document was to serve as a guide only and was not meant to inhibit or restrict the dialogue.

Some "Best Practice" subcommittee time was used to standardize interview method and style. This process provided comfort to members not as familiar with children and family services. Members then proceeded to conduct telephone interviews with the CEOs of the "Best Practice" agencies. As telephone interviews were completed, presentations to the Task Force were scheduled. These presentations introduced a wide range of structural models and operational designs of agency boards and stimulated creative dialogue as the group began to explore what could be learned and eventually incorporated.

The final activities in the process involved reviewing all findings and the formulation of Task Force recommendations for the Board of Directors.

By May 1996, following three months of work and seven meetings, the Board Restructuring Task Force had the following information in hand as it began to compile its recommendations:

1. Notes from the October 1995 Retreat, which expressed the general wishes of the Board.
2. The formal charge given to the Task Force by the Board.
3. The set of characteristics that the Task Force itself wished for the redesigned Board to have.
4. A literature search and discussion notes related to pertinent articles.
5. Completed questionnaires that described the practices of six other Boards of Directors from similar agencies.
6. The same questionnaire, describing the Center's own practice.

This information was critical to the legitimacy of the Task Force, to the eventual acceptance by the Board of its recommendations, and to the likely efficacy of the recommendations once they had been implemented. The process had been painstaking and admittedly tedious at times, but shortcuts would have undercut the force of the entire effort.

The Task Force developed its recommendations in the now familiar way: a period of open brainstorming was conducted that generated a sizable list of suggestions. These were then reviewed by the group with reference to the list of desired characteristics. Some rephrasing was incorporated, and redundancies were eliminated. The group finally approved ten specific recommendations (Appendix B). These specific recommendations address four chief areas:

Size of the Board. Several considerations were important. How big was too big for effective action? How small was too small to provide solid resource development capability? What number was needed to guarantee that the Board's multiple functions could be carried out? What was the limit of the Center's ability to provide individualized and meaningful experiences for the Directors?

The Task Force recommended reducing the maximum number for voting Directors from a potential of 50 to 25, with a minimum of 15. These voting Directors were to be called "Managing Directors." There were 32 active Directors at the time of the study. The Task Force, therefore, recommended that implementation of the reduction occur over two years, so that the vehicle of reduction would be natural attrition.

The Task Force also recommended that two other nonvoting categories of Director be established. "Associate Directors" would be a "friends of the agency" group that could include former Managing Directors, community members with interest but not the time to serve as Managing Directors, and people new to the agency who wanted to gain some experience before deciding to expand involvement. These Associate Directors could serve on ad hoc groups throughout the year, could attend all meetings, and complete orientation and training programs. The category might at once serve as a source of expert consultation, and as a pool of potential Managing Directors who have an advance body of experience with the Center.

The second category, Honorary Life Director, was to be composed of people from a variety of stations–volunteers, former staff members, former Board members–who have provided outstanding service to the Center over many years. As with the Associate Directors, Honorary Life Directors were to be nonvoting, but with broad access to the Center's work through ad hoc groups and unrestricted meeting attendance privileges.

Composition of the Board. The Task Force realized that the Board's membership must be composed so that it could perform at least three functions: represent the diversity of the community, gather resources, and provide technical expertise and consultation to the staff.

Consequently, its final recommendations contained guidelines for Board composition. The Task Force hoped that the new "Associate Director" category would compensate for any representational weaknesses that might exist in the "Managing Director" group at any point in time.

Action Format. How would the Board do its work? The Task Force concluded that fewer general meetings would suffice, provided that smaller, well-focused meetings took place more frequently. The Task Force further proposed increasing the role of the Executive Committee, specifying a larger number of meetings by this body to compensate for the reduced number of general meetings. It suggested reducing the number of standing committees from seven to four, while relying more heavily on the ad hoc groups, or task forces, that would meet to accomplish specific goals within limited periods. These ad hoc groups could be staffed by Directors and interested members of the community as appropriate. This model, the group hoped, would address the need expressed by Directors to be more involved in meaningful activity and less tied up in routine rubber-stamping. The Task Force also speculated that by allowing smaller groups of Directors to set their own meeting schedules, conflicts between Board schedules and personal schedules might be reduced in number.

Board-Executive Director Relationship. The Task Force recommended language intended to clarify the previous vaguely defined working relationship between the Board and the Executive Director. Three general areas of activity were defined in which Board approval would be required. The Task Force proposed language calling for Board approval around disposal or acquisition of significant assets, proposals for new services not clearly part of the Center's Mission, and proposals that might alter the Center's legal definition. The goal here was to assure that these critical functions remained under Board oversight, while giving the Executive Director sufficient latitude to manage Center operations efficiently. To assure competent Board governance, both content and process of the Executive Director's annual performance evaluation was addressed.

At the conclusion of its activities, the Task Force submitted the following proposal to the Board:

> The Board of Directors should form a task force to rewrite the Board *Bylaws* and its *Policies and Procedures*. The task force

should reorganize the existing material as appropriate and should incorporate the specific recommendations. . . .

The Board approved this recommendation unanimously at the last meeting of the year, disbanded the Board Restructuring Task Force, and established the *Bylaws* Revision Task Force. The *Bylaws* group was charged with incorporating the more specific restructuring recommendations into the Center's *Bylaws* and the Board's *Policies and Procedures*. The new group met through the summer and completed its work by the fall. On September 24, 1996, eleven months after the Retreat, the Board approved revisions that altered its fundamental structure.

EPILOGUE

The Board recently completed its second year of functioning under the new structure. With one year left before the new maximum limit becomes operational, the number of Directors has decreased to 27. There are 38 Associate Directors, six of whom have participated in task forces or on committees. Three of the six Managing Directors added over the course of two years have come from the Associate Director's category. The Nominating Committee has paid close attention to the recommendations concerning Board composition; two of the new Directors are from families that have received services through the Center, and others have brought specific expertise in the areas of education, health services, government, and managed care.

In addition to the four standing committees (Executive, Finance, Nominating, and Community Development and Fund Raising), the Board has formed seven task forces. One of these–Managed Care–has continued throughout the period. Others–Board Training, *Bylaws* Update, and Program Report Review, for example–have executed their charges and disbanded. As previously noted above, both the task forces and committees have offered opportunity for Associate Directors to contribute directly to the Center within the constraints of their available time.

Board attendance at Managing Directors' meetings is up 10% over that prior to the restructuring. On the other hand, the most specific criticism to date has concerned the reduction of meetings to five per year. Some Directors, particularly those not actively engaged in task forces, have complained that they have felt more distant from the Center, and that if they miss a single meeting, they find themselves hopelessly out of touch. This issue will require attention.

It is certainly too early to say what the ultimate fate of the various reforms will be, however, overall initial indications are encouraging. The Board is scheduled to conduct its self-review this year, and the format will be designed to evaluate the changes presented.

DISCUSSION

1. The simple facts of a Board's defined structure are extremely, although not supremely, important. Structure cannot make magic–magic requires dedicated and competent people. But a poor structure can diminish the efforts of the best Board members. Structures that do not account for changing circumstance and demand can inhibit rather than facilitate the most well-intentioned efforts.

    Boards and staff must realize that the unreviewed accretion of policy and practice over periods of years can lead eventually to petrification, the last quality needed in an age that appears to demand speed and flexibility from nonprofit organizations. Regular review and occasional overhaul of structure may be essential.

2. The process of change described above can be summarized briefly: the Board members expressed their needs and desires; the working group described what the Board was currently doing; the group looked carefully at what other Boards across the country were doing; it studied relevant literature; and finally, the thoughts of its individual members were articulated and spread out for all Task Force members to see. These were condensed, phrased as recommendations, and returned to the Board.

    The composition of the planning group is an important part of the process. It need not be–indeed, probably should *not* be–comprised exclusively of current Board members. Former Board members, who carry the Board's history with them, are essential, as are staff members, who have a realistic sense of the demands of Board administration. Visionaries, who may or may not be current Board members, are, of course, necessary to spark the process.

3. The "Associate Director" category–those special friends of the Center–seems particularly important for several reasons, and others contemplating Board reorganization are referred to it. The category makes possible varieties of professional expertise on a voluntary basis, provides a training-incubation period for prospective Managing Directors (so important for today's complex multiple service organization), allows for broad involvement by many who do not have the time to serve as Managing Directors, and provides personpower for Board functions that is not available through the streamlined Managing Director group.

Associate status allows a Board to compensate for the sacrifices that attend streamlining. While smaller Managing Boards may be necessary for the type of intense participation and flexibility needed for response to change and competition, the community nonprofit, nevertheless, still requires broad support and access from a large number of citizens. Access to Center process as a "special friend" constitutes an invitation and opportunity for such involvement.

4. The "Honorary Life Director" category allows for the expression of appreciation to community members and former staff members who have served the Center with distinction for many years. This category provides the benefits of the "Associate Director" class and also preserves the Center's "institutional memory."

REFERENCES

Bowen, W. G. (September-October 1994). When a Business Leader Joins a Nonprofit Board. *Harvard Business Review*, 38-43.

Firstenberg, P. B., and Malkiel, B. G. (Fall 1994). The Twenty-First Century Boardroom: Who Will Be in Charge? *Sloan Management Review*, 27-35.

Herzlinger, R. E. (July-August 1994). Effective Oversight: A Guide for Nonprofit Directors. *Harvard Business Review*, 52-60.

Johnson, D. W., Smale, J. G., and *Harvard Business Review* Interviews with Alan J. Patricof, Sir Denys Henderson, and Bernard Marcus (March-April 1995). Can an empowered board and a strong CEO co-exist? Redraw the Line Between the Board and the CEO. *Harvard Business Review*, 153-164.

Lasell, D. M., and Jensen, C. M. (1992). Bridging the Gap Between Nonprofit and For-Profit Board Members. Nonprofit Government Series, National Center for Nonprofit Boards, Washington, DC.

Lorsch, J. W. (January-February 1995). Empowering the Board. *Harvard Business Review*, 107-117.

Taylor, B. E., Chait, R. P., Holland, T P. (September-October 1996). The New Work of the Nonprofit Board. *Harvard Business Review*, 36-46.
Williams, L. D. (1994). Family and Children's Center, Inc., Multiple-Corporation Organizational Model, unpublished paper.

APPENDIX A:
DESIRED CHARACTERISTICS
OF REDESIGNED BOARD

- The Board will be committed to the Agency culture and mission.
- The Board will be entrepreneurial, alert to change and opportunity, and capable of imaginative and timely action.
- The Board will have access to information. It will bring to the Agency information from government, private industry, and recipients of service.
- The Board will have clear roles for each member. Everyone will know what they contribute as individuals, and as a group, to the operation of the Agency.
- The Board will manage conflict openly and constructively. There will be free exchange of views, and a clear path to decision.
- The Board will have political influence, and use that judiciously on behalf of the Agency and its clients.
- The Board will have access to service funders, whether public or private, and will use that access judiciously on behalf of the Agency and its clients.
- The Board will possess pertinent "industry" expertise, by virtue of membership and training.
- The Board will be capable of raising money for the Agency.

APPENDIX B:
SPECIFIC RECOMMENDATIONS OF THE TASK FORCE

1. Reduce membership, as current Directors rotate off the Board, to a maximum of 25 and a minimum of 15.
2. Specify the following guidelines for Board composition. The Board membership will:
   a. Reflect the diversity of the community and the variety of groups and individuals affected by Agency activity.

    b. Give the Agency access to the political and business processes that affect its ability to realize its Mission.

    c. Provide support for the Agency's efforts to develop resources that will help it advance the Mission.

    d. Provide oversight of policy that is based on identification with Agency Mission and Values, awareness of Agency operations, and specific expertise in particular areas of Agency activity.

3. Redefine Associate membership to include persons who have not been affiliated with the Agency previously. Provide for non-voting participation in Board activities. The Nominating Committee will administer the Associate membership.

4. The Executive Committee will consist of the Officers of the Board and the Committee Chairs. The Executive Committee will meet monthly and as needed to process agendas set by the Board President and the Executive Director. The Executive Committee will authorize the development of task forces as needed.

5. Task forces will be time-limited and focused on clearly defined jobs. Membership may consist of Board members, Associates, Agency staff and invited members of the general community.

6. The full Board will meet five times per year, and as needed. Agendas will be set by the Executive Committee.

7. There will be three standing committees in addition to the Executive Committee that will meet regularly and as needed: Finance, Community Development and Fund Raising, and Nominating. Finance will continue its current functions. Community Development and Fund Raising will access private funding and will establish relationships for the Agency within the donor community. Nominating will retain traditional duties involving designation of candidates for the Board and its offices, and will add the administration of the Associate membership. Functions formerly managed by the Program Committee will be managed through the annual education plan and through special task forces.

8. Annual task forces will be convened to perform the following jobs: review of governing documents and developing the annual Board education plan.

9. A committee consisting of the Board President, two Officers, and two other Board members will review the performance and compensation of the Executive Director. The committee will also establish new annual goals in conjunction with the Executive Director. The committee may confer with the Agency's Human Resources Director as necessary during the evaluation process.

10. The following language is proposed concerning the Board's delegation of authority to the Executive Director:

    The Board of Directors delegates to the Executive Director the authority to operate the Agency to forward the Mission. Board approval in advance is required for:

    a. Proposals to acquire or dispose of significant Agency assets, as defined by an annual resolution of the Board.
    b. The development of programming or business activity not described in the Agency Mission.
    c. Proposals to amend the Agency's legal definition.

    The Executive Director will keep the Board fully informed of all Agency activity so that the Board can exercise its oversight responsibility.

Index

Accountability
    of CEOs, 1
    financial, 25-27
    service, 27
Acquisitions, role of boards and CEOs
    and, 9-11
Austin, Nancy, 64-65

Blanchard, Ken, 65
Board matrix, 8,18
Board members, nonprofit
    diversity of, xvii-xviii
    executive directors and, xviii
    roles of, xviii
    as strategists, 5-7
    traditional, xii-xiv
Boards, nonprofit. *See also* Nonprofit
    organizations
    as advocates for change, 13
    change process of, for nonprofits,
      77-87
    continuing education of, 58-60
    corporate model of, 70-71
    developing effective, 52
    developing strategic advantage
      with composition of, 7-9
    disagreement and, xix
    educating, for fund raising, 44
    fiduciary responsibility of, 22-23
    fund raising role of, 46
    governance and policy action of, 41
    harnessing talents of, 2-3
    leadership of, in communities,
      11-13
    legal obligations of, 22-23
    long range planning and, 44-47
    maximizing relations with CEOs,
      13-16
    mergers and, 9-11

multi-corporation model of, 70-76
needs of, for effective performance,
    3
negligence and, 23
responsibilities of, 52-53
risk management and, 21,27
roles and functions of, 21-22
skills of, 2
staffs and, 44-46
strategic affiliations and, 9-11
tasks of, xix
traditional model of, 70
traditional orientation and training
    of, 43-44
training of, 32-34

Capitated payments, 55,56-57
CEOs *See* Chief executive officers
    (CEOs)
Chait, Richard P., 2,5
Change, xvii-xviii
    boards as advocates for, 13
    process of, for boards, 77-87
Chief executive officers (CEOs)
    accountability of, 67-68
    boards and, xviii
    as clock builders, 66-67
    continuing education of boards and,
      59
    evaluation of, 15-16
    harnessing talents of boards and,
      2-3
    maximizing relations with boards,
      13-16
    preparing boards for strategic
      planning and, 6-7
    role of, in mergers and strategic
      affiliations, 10-11
    training and professional
      development of, 14-15